Evesonderism

EVESONDERISM

Living the Story
of the Art of
Narrative Medicine

JEAN ROBEY, MD

Afterword by Dr. Marcia Reynolds

Evesonderism
Living the Story of the Art of Narrative Medicine

For information about this title or to order other books and/or electronic media, contact the publisher:

Ethos of Medicine
https://ethosofmedicine.wordpress.com

ISBNs:
979-8-9999568-2-8 (hardcover)
979-8-9999568-0-4 (softcover)
979-8-9999568-1-1 (eBook)

Printed in the United States of America

Cover design: Jaxen Robey
and Interior design: 1106 Design

To my father, Giang Vo, for his insight, preparation, and bravery to come to America, my mother, De Vo, for her courage to leave her home and constantly make a better one for her family, and the two families that sponsored us to America, the Roaches and the LeMasters.

Contents

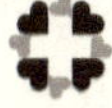

Foreword

By Bryce Palmer University of Arizona College of Medicine—Phoenix, Class of 2028

I met Dr. Jean Robey shortly after matriculating into medical school. She quickly evolved into a Narrative Medicine mentor and thought-provoking friend. Her personal and meaningful approach to doctoring embodies the reasons I chose to pursue medicine.

As a first-year medical student, my training is focused on developing the clinical skills crucial to doctoring. Although my enrollment into certificate of distinction tracts help me to focus on other aspects of medicine, doctoring can easily become mechanical. Dr. Robey helped me find meaning in patient care beyond a diagnosis. Instrumentally, she introduced me to the word *sonder*—the profound realization that every person we encounter has a life as vivid and complex as our own. This word captures how I wish to interact with my patients. Instead of checklists and cases, Dr. Robey reminds me that each patient carries stories worth hearing.

During my undergraduate training, I was fortunate to be trained as a professional coach. I enjoyed coaching and the clarity it could help those receiving coaching achieve. I came to medical school with a revised dream: to integrate coaching values and medicine to create a more charitable approach to patient care. Coaching teaches me how powerful it is to listen deeply, ask meaningful questions, and honor people's unique journeys. Narrative Medicine honors the time-honored heart of doctoring while drawing out the life-shaping stories we hear as doctors using coach-like skills. Together, Dr. Robey and I found an intriguing thought to coach physicians in training and eventually coach the coach-like skills used in exercising Narrative Medicine to achieve the best physician-patient relationships and outcomes.

In *Evesonderism: Living the Story of the Art of Narrative Medicine*, Dr. Robey shares moments when personal narratives and medicine meet. Her collection of stories shares common sentiments and unique details. They teach through storytelling, story-seeking as a methodology for doctoring effectively. Here, the work of doctoring becomes increasingly meaningful and personal. Dr. Robey brings decades of experience, humanity, and bright vision to her practice. These are not just medical stories but sentiments that beg us to pause, listen, and ask: What does it mean to be a successful doctor? Is it a teachable communication style based on complex things we can tap into concretely?

The story "Dialogue" particularly portrayed this for me. In this narrative we experience how coaching bridged the space between humanity and medicine. While knowledgeable of procedures and biology, Dr. Robey also recognized human elements of care. She created a space, amid a chaotic, tragic, pre-op room, that empowered a grieving wife to navigate a deeply personal moment with her injured husband. Narrative Medicine, in this moment, allowed for a deeper understanding of how clinical medicine fits into the larger tapestry of a couple's lives. Narrative Medicine exacted the best attributes of human contact via doctoring.

To you, the reader: Whether you are a first-year medical student just beginning your journey like me, or a seasoned physician with decades of experience like Dr. Robey, these stories have the power to deepen and transform the way we practice medicine through a side journey into stories and empathy felt by narrative immersion. Narrative Medicine invites both newcomers and veterans to connect with the heart of our work, seeing patients as people and not just cases. We are bridging a past older than ourselves and a future that will carry on long after us. I hope these stories remind you, as they remind me, that the best medicine begins with truly seeing people for who they are and as complex as we each are.

Introduction

We begin at the infinite. We begin at *sonder*. Sonder is the surprisingly underappreciated word to represent the profound feeling of realizing that everyone, including strangers passing in the street, has a life as complex as one's own, which they are constantly living.

Evesonderism is a neologism encompassing living in this state of awareness.

If we begin at the infinite, we arrive at the conclusion that could encompass the infinite. We arrive at narratives.

Many orders draw from medical ethics, communication, and humanism to exact and teach the skill sets needed to best preserve the finest, most fundamental yet evolving considerations of medical engagements between physician and patient. One such practice is Narrative Medicine. Narrative Medicine maintains that the breath of humanistic qualities that tell a story meet best the medical nexus. The patient's narrative becomes the point of origin to consider and to navigate along and merge with medical advice for a more perfect physician and patient journey. A narrative focus employs various facets including close reading.

Close reading borrows from the practice of literary criticism to help hone elements of attentive, critical, and careful reading. Close reading in literature treats the literary body as its own entity and seeks to understand it as if it is alive with "massive, and subtle, impact."[1] Close reading is a complex skill that many aspiring and practicing physicians already exhibit. It requires closely watching and sensing all aspects of a situation—the words, body language, setting, hierarchy, assumptions, choice, priority, pauses, context, companions, hesitations, ease, discomfort, beliefs, manipulations, emotions, eye contact, utterances, shifts, unrest, and relief, to say the least, in an engagement. In literary criticism, the exercise of close reading analyzes the words, descriptions, context, and supporting and evolving chapters in a concrete way so that a literary critic can discover a well-formed character, motive, plot, and thematic statement.

Applying close reading to doctoring elegantly transfers all those applicable nuances to the physician-patient relationship. The patient's life, an ongoing narrative, is the platform a physician is suddenly thrusted into and trusted with. At that often intrusive juncture, the physician is to contribute unique and critical insights. The patient cannot therefore be just a predetermined equation subjected to a generic, algorithmic assessment.

Narrative Medicine borrows from established and even flawed literary criticism to have concrete approaches to practice. A practicing narrative physician would employ many of the conscious and subconscious attributes found in immersing into a well-written piece of literature. A physician practicing Narrative Medicine essentially reads a patient as a story and adds to that story the role of the engrossed reader, providing suitable medical advice, delivered with the most accepted and reconciled ways to communicate to that individual, to be fully useful and most natural to the patient before them. Flawed aspects of literary criticism prove also the power and accuracy of using such skills found in literary

---

1 Cleanth Brooks and Robert Penn Warren, *Understanding Poetry* (New York: Holt, Rinehart and Winston, 1976), xiii.

criticism. At times the reader cannot fully appreciate a work of literature because of cultural bias and ignorance. Specifically, close reading in Narrative Medicine can be proof that bias and ignorance alter the potential engagement for a physician and patient. In the very flaws are the proof that we are a widely diverse social creatures who need unique and broad experiences to best appreciate each other. An argument can be made for the necessity of diversifying experiences and providers to best encompass all the possible people who become patients, needing help and fundamental derivation despite differences.

Why it took twenty-five years . . .

Many people encouraged me to publish my stories, and for a decade I waited to. I felt I was missing some understanding of the power of my stories and the beauty that they can invite to appreciate unique and often relatable experiences. The purpose of the stories seemed inappropriately singular until events in time unfolded my understanding.

My deepest hopes are that by combining a compilation of inspired stories that my years of being a physician have gifted me as examples alongside the concrete model for practicing Narrative Medicine first laid out by Dr. Rita Charon,[2] I can teach the practice of Narrative Medicine as a state of engagement that can lead to preserving the best aspects of excellent and rewarding doctoring. Everything erosive and divisive in society seems to threaten this important ability to connect and to understand how to connect. Additionally, coaching the physician to fuller self-awareness and then teaching the additional coach-like skills to execute the physician's role to fully find, guide, bridge, and profit the patient is the quintessential encapsulation of the future of medical training that best preserves the ethos of medicine. It is the art of medicine best elucidated by the art of observing and appreciating

---

2 Rita Charon, et al. *The Principles and Practice of Narrative Medicine* (New York: Oxford University Press, 2017).

the art of humans. It is the story of the art of medicine. I have finally understood the narrative of my joy and journey as a physician and the ongoing collection of stories I amass as the pattern of humanity unfolded intimately in my office.

How it began . . .

I paused my passion for writing when I entered the rigors of getting into and proceeding through medical school, residency, and fellowship. Many artist-scientist-philosopher types paused such things, feeling that the science of medicine is so powerful a mistress that all one's time and attention must be devoted to acquiring that perfect truth. My passion for storytelling and writing returned to me as a desperate life raft. I found after exiting training and beginning my career as a private-practice nephrologist that I became without hope or clarity. There I was five years into my career and I was bored and disconnected from the very real and very tangible celestial bodies invited into private and trusting engagements. I started writing about little things that mattered, and whether the striking things birthed their own need for storytelling or my quest became to find details for storytelling I cannot tell since they became one in the same. Long before the vocabulary existed, I was already intrigued by details and logged them, but never did I think the details of people's universes onto themselves would present a teachable pursuit, a highly desirable element to preserve, and a life raft for me and all. It was years later that I found the definition that declared my practice Narrative Medicine with an actual framework that perfectly deduced what my practice had been constructed thus far instinctually. This exacting insight invited the overwhelming joy that the art of medicine could be reproduced with rapid clarity.

How it now is . . .

This collection has four aspects. The first is a series of my short stories and poems that exemplify close reading in action. These stories are a fraction of my collection but represent my own evolution as a physician and provide the methodology to teach Narrative Medicine. The actualization of stories proves they exist in constant materialization. The reading of stories of doctoring is the best way to teach, much like watching the perfect three-point shot indirectly synthesizes the complex explanations that lose feel for piecemealed instructions. The second is a stewardship. I explored many potential aspects of my journey with medical writing and eventually met Bryce Palmer. Bryce Palmer graciously and skillfully supplied the foreword. Bryce has been coaching for some time and has a love for coaching, but his original love was medicine. His perspective at the beginning of medical training is so very far from my twenty-five years of practicing medicine but from an angle already committed to and experienced with coaching. We will be better physicians, he and I, for the expertise we give each other as we move along the same timeline toward each other. As we arrive toward each other's narratives, we see the exact hallmark of close reading as it is being written for us both. It is our differing vantage points along a career path converging that proves we can sustain the ethos of medicine with passionate conviction rewarded by exact execution.

The third aspect is a sample reflection written by my daughter, Jade Robey. She has lived with my bias all her life, and as she enters medicine and learns close reading and the value it brings to medicine and her own devotion as a physician, she materializes the model that can sustain the future of medicine and doctoring. I am amazed at her thoughts about what impression she was left with that will shape her empathy and her delivery of medicine for years to come. Would you not want such an insightful physician providing the medical elements to best suit your narrative?

Finally, there is an afterword by Dr. Marcia Reynolds,[3] who is a brilliant and naturally gifted life coach. I asked her to speak, as she has in

3 Marcia Reynolds, *Outsmart Your Brain*, second edition (Covisioning, 2017).

many of her own books, about the value of coaching and thereby lay out the things it is, but also discuss why doctoring is not coaching but has coach-like skills we can thus teach and also effectively utilize in practicing Narrative Medicine to the betterment of patient engagements. I met with Dr. Reynolds many times to share my theory about the essential ethos of medicine and its best instruction. She wholeheartedly validated the need for meaningful physician-patient engagement, having, like many, her own examples of being a patient and feeling disconnected. She also embraced the methodology of practicing Narrative Medicine to achieve the more ideal connection driven by focus on personal narratives. Dr. Reynolds affirmed the coachlike skills doctors use and agreed to the need and ready opportunity to coach those skills to aspiring physicians.

By adding the elements of Narrative Medicine, most importantly coaching close reading for physician development, the doctor can doctor with a whole unadulterated heart, like a reader has for a beloved and evolving character on a journey in a book. The physician can also persevere when coaching becomes advice, measuring exactly the value of giving it along the power of a story needing to be told perfectly.

In summary, Narrative Medicine means a kind of engrossed engagement with a patient. We know this engagement by our own personal experience with books and characters in books. As readers of books we immerse into storylines. Doctors are not life coaches. They immerse to coach but also specifically to advise, which means they must go into a personal storyline and insert perfectly the medical advice. By clear comparison, coaching is a parallel engagement, and doctoring pushes the boundaries of coaching into a place where people are also advised. A perfectly told story should flow medically as well. Perfect doctoring should exact the same inspired excellence in storytelling and never betray the patient's theme and evolution. Coaching the elements of Narrative Medicine and its coach-like skills is the forefront of teaching the art of medicine. In this understanding, framework, and mentorship, the patient remains the center of the sonder. The physician's journey, like mine, becomes itself a story that embraces sonder; one of evesonderism. Why would I not gift that insight early to an aspiring physician or heal one who is tiring?

It has been a long time waiting to best understand the potential value of stories born of the very privileged moments in doctoring that inspire and relate us to one another. I share this journey with you, the reader, to invite it as a part of your narrative moving forward. The potential of the totality of years of human insight from suffering and loss can best be honored if you help carry all of it with purpose forward. Look for a physician subscribing to Narrative Medicine or be a physician who practices Narrative Medicine and save and elevate for all time the time-honored relationship of physician-patient.

A word of caution . . .

I once watched a YouTube video in which Dr. Rita Charon, considered by all to be the Mother of Narrative Medicine, began to discuss Narrative Medicine and apologized for seeming like she was talking only of death. The profound common ground of being mortal proves that in facing death we have much to reconcile as our narratives are forced into very sharp focus. I know my stories will seem often similarly tragic, but that is because they are tied together by the crucible of reflection and inflection points that include an absolute guarantee like death and the testaments that define the moments before it. Otherwise, each story is a unique journey like all of you are embracing each day.

The last unique contribution to this book includes my son, Jaxen, who designed the cover, which has been on my mind for so many years. Since childhood, I saw each of us in a vast ocean only capable of being in individual boats that could only be floating by or at best tied together but never would we be in the same boat.

The truths that became self-evident in years of not studying medicine but in thriving while witnessing and orchestrating symphonies with universes I called my patients are woven here room after room. My patients call me their doctor, and I dedicate this book to them. I thank deeply my parents, who first believed in my passions; my siblings, who protected me and supported me; my husband Kirk, who finds me wonderfully odd but lovely all the same; my daughter Jade, who will one day embrace the growing intellect and profound emotions of doctoring herself; and my son Jaxen, who taught me the word I have been looking my entire life to share when he spoke of sonder.

Finally, thank you to the readers of my humbly offered collection. I confess, there were times when I had no readers, yet, I was so grateful that the words holding onto a sentiment and soul were written and not lost, let alone read and digested. Readers are poignant to stories, for at least there are reasons for the suffering—often painful but ultimately beautiful derivations that inspire them.

Disclaimer

Please be aware of the potential triggers in the stories curated. The collection often speaks of loss and end of life issues, even suicide, rape, drug addition, and child death. The essential nuance of Narrative Medicine often reflects at crucial moments that accumulate as we are threatened by illness, death, or loss. It is recommended readers read stories over time and to limit the reading of many at one sitting. It is not sadness that is collected here. Sadness is only a reflection of greatness ending. The bittersweet, the irony in being mortal is what I hope readers will appreciate about evesonderism.

The Retainer

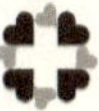

Early on, having patients come in to see me as their doctor was a honeymoon thrill. I had to measure up to prior opinions and styles. I had to develop a style, my style. Honestly, I was faking authority till I had any. I was trying to make good on all that training I invested in and others invested in. One day I was a fellow and then the next day I was an attending, and the proverbial buck was supposed to stop at my high heels.

I inherited a practice of two hundred patients. They were shifty and leery at first. A few I was grateful for were nonchalant, somehow accustomed to abandonment and reorganization.

Of those I inherited who were cautious and critical were Agnes and Lester.

Agnes would walk her husband Lester in each time. She was organized and meticulous.

"Lester, sit here," she would direct.

They were both my patients. She had high blood pressure. He had the higher creatinine and thus the worse prognosis. Their combined age was 174, and their combined renal function was less than 60 percent.

Lester was a charmer and a very sweet man who loved well his children and wife. Agnes was a proper mother. Together they had fourteen children. Many were nurses. All were in their forties to sixties.

"We always wanted our kids to have two Christmas presents each year," Lester said one visit, eyes mischievous. "One year Agnes and I wrapped one sleeve and one shoe for one kid, the other sleeve and the other shoe for one kid, the vest and a toy for one kid!" The two laughed heartily. I burst with laughter!

I passed by their sons at work, not knowing for years they were nurses in the ICU.

Agnes fed Lester seaweed tablets daily, and his creatinine would inch back. "Chlorophyll—a powerful antioxidant," described the inserts. I said, "Sure!" Seeing no issues.

Meanwhile, Agnes had terribly labile blood pressure. Her ultrasound showed renal asymmetry, and I had recommended renal angiogram to evaluate and stent what looked like renal artery stenosis. She said firmly, "No." Agnes was here only "to be sure Lester didn't get into trouble," she clarified.

One day, Agnes went into hypertensive crisis. Her blood pressure shot up and suddenly her kidneys shut down. She found herself abruptly on dialysis. Shocked and confused because Lester had always been the sicker one, she mentally collapsed. Wasn't he the one with a prior bypass now thready? Wasn't he the one with 25 percent kidney function?

Broadsided by catastrophic events, she was catatonic. Her sons and daughters were at the bedside as sons and daughters, not nurses.

She was eventually discharged home to perform outpatient dialysis.

The daughters would take turns coming into my office with their father, now the new wardens, or they would sit chairside at dialysis with their mother as trusted allies. Lester's visits were uneventful. Agnes agonized. "Mom is very cold at dialysis." "Mom is not eating." "Mom is so tired after dialysis." "Mom was confused this morning." Agnes took to wearing ski gear to dialysis—a huge puffy pair of ski pants and a puffy jacket that swallowed her up.

For a year I dialyzed her and tried to outfit the world according to Agnes.

Eventually to lessen the needs and shine more light on his wife, Lester came to see me on his own.

One day Lester came while holding a small brown paper bag. The bag had a strange grease stain on the bottom that crawled up one side of the bag.

I was busy writing the note in his chart as he sat quietly. I outlined the history and medications and labs. Paper charts were still widely used, but guidelines for charting were becoming more extensive. To keep on task, I had to prep a little as patients waited. I was busy, head down, scribbling.

"I have been thinking," Lester said.

"Uh-huh," I said, not looking up, still writing.

"I was thinking," he continued as he took a deep breath, "if I stop my Plavix and aspirin and then Agnes stops her dialysis, maybe we can die together," Lester said.

I stopped writing but didn't look up. I stared at the paper for just a second to absorb what he had said. Then I looked up. Our eyes met.

He extended his left arm and placed the brown bag on the table.

"I brought these," he said.

I looked at the greasy bag on the table.

I opened it and looked in.

There were a dozen doughnut holes in the bag. I smiled hugely and took one of the doughnuts out and began eating it. I rolled out from behind my desk and over to his chair while holding the bag. Still chewing, I casually offered him a doughnut hole from the bag too. He reached in eagerly to accept a naughty thing a doctor gave him.

"That's an interesting plan. Have you told your kids?" I chewed.

"No," he chewed.

I swallowed and grabbed another doughnut hole. "Well, it won't work," I admitted.

Lester chewed slower than me, having nowhere to go, and halfheartedly shrugged. "It was just an idea," he smiled.

"Thanks for the doughnut holes," I said, offering the greasy bag back.

"There's more where those came from." He winked. "I want to keep you on retainer," he said, pushing the offering back.

I burst into laughter again! "Lawyers are raking it in to stand and be ready to defend a client. Meanwhile, I'm getting fat on greasy doughnut holes." I shook my head, disappointed. "You are a charmer!" I exclaimed and took the bag back.

Even on dialysis, Agnes would still close each monthly round to ask that I "okay" the seaweed pills for Lester.

"I'll tell him, Agnes," I would promise.

Agnes took a turn. True to literature, she didn't last much more than a year, given age alone.

Lester arrived in my office a month later on queue.

"Hi," he said.

"You okay?" I hugged.

"Yeah," he said, sorted and calm.

He sat and I gave a pause before launching into the visit and our fifteen-minute agenda.

"Hey," he said, "I have something to ask you."

I readied myself and said, "Okay, go."

Lester had been conversing with an old friend from high school for the last weeks. She lived in New York. She was coming out to see him.

"I want your permission," he asked as politely and respectfully as if I were his mother.

I smiled my huge doughnut hole smile and asked first, "Did you ask your kids?"

Lester said, "Yeah, they all don't mind, but you knew Agnes and I think if you said it was okay . . ."

My god. I guess at some point Agnes became my ward, and I became her proxy. I began to see the fullness of the buck stopping at my feet.

"Sir, Lester, my dear friend. Agnes would want you to be happy." I hugged him long and hard.

He hugged me back.

The story goes that the old acquaintance came out for a visit, but being herself older and not well, she got sick and was hospitalized. She eventually returned home to New York. Shortly after the visit, I heard that Lester died himself. I wondered if he had executed his little plan to stop Plavix and aspirin and let his tenuous bypass close, but it didn't matter. I like to think he merely died calmly, happily having loved hard and often laughing.

I can't eat a doughnut hole without thinking of being on a retainer for a greater calling than algorithms and mandates and outcomes. I am tempted each year to wrap fragments of gifts for my two children and laugh when they open them with a string attached, hoping the jacket or the shoes are theirs. I put on ski gear each winter and hope Agnes is plenty warm wherever she is. I respect the life-giving chlorophyll that offered control and solace to a woman caring for her husband. Lastly, I think love and romance happen even at eighty-eight years of age. Love is the retainer.

♥

Dialogue

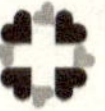

They say to not start a story with dialogue. The thrust of disorientation of who is speaking, where they are, and why they are there will put off the reader. Oh, the precious reader lurking on the other side of words on pages, hoping for a glance at something so utterly rich, a bit private and a bit scary to use as escape into the very present elsewhere.

"You take the wife aside and tell her we are getting the OR ready. You get her to sign those consents and explain the surgery, but be sure to explain more so the risk after surgery. I'll take the team to get the OR prepped and to round on the rest. Put a central line in him. Twenty minutes, Jean, it's all she's got to wrap up a lifetime," the chief said without even looking at me as he fluttered on the keyboard, ordering various things and charting. Then he left with a team in tow. The trauma bay stayed a disheveled mess with little litterings everywhere.

I had long since grown to hate the little pieces of garbage all over the floor in some haphazard proof of our incompetence to control cleanly chaos. Every day the trauma bay doors flung open and ruined order, and the cleansing smell of disinfectant was reapplied. I wished someone would come clean the bay now so things would start to be orderly again and help sort my thoughts like perfectly lined saline bags, bulbous and ready to spike. I knew the better thing to hope was that the wife would arrive soon so that the twenty minutes she had—we had—would not be wasted en route. I knew the better thing to pray was that the bay stay private, and that no other trauma would break the moments to come from twenty precious minutes barely allocated.

Six months of being a surgical intern, desperate to impress and learn, grueling for hours each day, day after day, makes for a kind of exponential competence that is part thrusted and part trusted. I had grown at ease with lines, developing a system to be self-sufficient and self-contained. I would systematically set up my kit in a way that let the guide wires stay readily deployable, and I made sure all medications were laid drawn and accessible with one quick hand off to myself. I arranged everything so perfectly that in the quiet of a room alone with a patient I could secure a line, and no one would even know I had been there and gone, tempting them to yell at me for not having done the line. I found a way to expeditiously contain the guide wire after using it by stuffing it into the unplunged syringe. Legendarily, when I was finished and cleaned up, one fellow intern thought my kit was unused. I found the process meditative, as I leaned into the exactness and the fluidity of every movement.

Six months of being a surgical intern, in which I was desperate to learn techniques and executions, did not exactly perfect simultaneously talking or balancing facts with comfort and compassion. It was scarier to approach a wife, a husband, a mother, a father, a child than to cut with a fresh sharp blade the skin and guide a device into the vein.

She was softly led to the hallway just before the trauma bay. Oddly, the short passageway was empty of people, and beyond that the nurses' desk was unmanned with them all tending to some other patients. She met me and her eyes were swollen and her face a bit plastic. Shock was a shawl over her skin, and the pores retreated for fear of feeling the real air and the reality of words I was unleashing like cuts from a sharper scalpel upon her flesh.

"Your husband was brought in just hours ago. He was in the bucket of the crane on the truck that hoisted the workers up to the power line. There was some water at the bottom of the bucket. He was working on the power line and there was a surge. That surge was massive given the bit of water he stood in, and that exposure has led to a severe and significant injury."

I paused to brace her and myself, feeling suddenly the infinite inadequacy of myself for my role. I could practice for a hundred years as a physician, yet telling bad news will always be the humbled trepidation I have mused in some vast wing of my subconsciousness. My ancillary brain spun around to think of how I, so small and irrelevant, was duty-bound to tell her all the details and get her somehow to shake out of shock to sign and capture the best of what was left possible to do. I felt like a cautious fool.

She waited and I took a deeper breath. "Are you okay right now? Can I trust you to be strong while I detail a few things?" I asked first.

She nodded anxiously to hear but did not fully understand the drama of asking permission to tell.

I braced us both and started again up the thick underbrush and mosquito-laden jungle of torturous details. It was getting hotter and hotter as I spoke and felt faint at times. "Your husband suffered a massive surge. What that does is damage all muscles instantly. They begin to swell, and we must release the skin and lining around the muscles to help the muscles not pressurize and become choked off from blood supply." She nodded, accepting this plan, but I pressed deeper into the dark parts of the jungle. "Your husband's exposure was very severe, and the electricity took the flesh right off both of his legs," I forced out.

"What do you mean?" she managed.

I took a deeper breath and wrung my face to reset the creases. My usual optimism was betrayed by truth as my voice cracked and my shoulders slumped. I felt small in the suddenly oversized white coat. Authority fell like a Hollywood studio façade and there we both were, vulnerable.

"The surge," I began again, adjusting my posture to invite confidence and shield me from the supernova-like pain the wife would feel. "The surge," I repeated, stuck like a child fascinated by rot that overtook a log in the jungle, "it burned off all the flesh on his legs clear to the bones and cauterized the pelvis instantly. Please don't look at all. It will never leave you, this image."

She peered into the trauma bay and saw his sneakers sticking out from under the blanket.

"I see his shoes, though," she pondered, conflicted with a reality told and one that was not him when they kissed goodbye that morning.

"He has fused with his shoes, and his pants are tattered and shredded, but his upper half is still intact. He is miraculously awake, talking." I stopped for her to focus on the last, worried she would need me to abuse her with repetition.

"He is awake?" she blinked.

"Yes. He is awake. He is unaware of what has happened exactly. He is calm. He is not in pain. He knows he is at the hospital but only because there was an accident and some commotion. He is stable but," I braced her, "not for long. He must go to surgery immediately, and we only have ten to fifteen minutes before they take him."

She nodded, eager to see him.

I stuttered through the consents and the details, asking her to just sign as the surgery was multiple fasciotomies and a complex hemicorporectomy that few could survive. "They take the whole lower half," I shortened. As she signed slowly, half present, I added, "The damage to muscle in other areas will very likely postoperatively cause a severe acidosis and collapse of all systems in hours. This was a last-ditch effort to be doing anything when nothing is likely to work. What I need you to focus on is just being with him because that is a gift and he is oddly, miraculously awake. He is in a state of shock, but he is aware and experiencing things so please just talk gently to him," I guided her. "Ma'am," I said as she started away from me and toward her husband, "let me be clear. He will not survive this. Please be with him knowing this."

"What do I," she stuttered now too, "say to him? What am I supposed to talk about?"

We stood for ten precious seconds and then I asked, "Did you have any plans coming up?"

She inventoried their lives, rapidly recalling a movie he had asked her to earlier in the week.

"We were supposed to maybe go to the movies tonight," she offered.

"Talk about the plans you had tentatively for tonight. The movie, maybe dinner before," I handed back.

"Does he know he's dying?" she braved.

"I didn't tell him exactly, but also I don't think he can compute or recall things we all have said. He seems pleasantly stuck in a kind of euphoria due to the shock. I haven't made excessive efforts to get dooming details across. It seemed cruel and unnecessary," I apologized. "People know unsaid things. I left it vague so it cannot fill the room and hide you," I explained.

She nodded and we made our way back to him alone in the trauma bay, a blanket drawn up past his chest and the monitor overhead quieted but steady. She circled to his head, which was turned to the left, and smiled to see him looking so normal lying on the gurney.

"Hi, Babe," she whispered.

He smiled back and replied, "Hi, Hon. I didn't know you were here."

They took to whispering about the day, and she started immediately asking which movie he picked. He was excited about seeing *Star Wars: The Phantom Menace* and she rolled her eyes and teased that it was her turn to pick. They planned where they would have dinner, and she asked him to split their dish so she could eat two meals, being good on her diet, and they laughed.

I set up my central line tray off to the side and draped his head and neck, and I made a tent that partitioned me from her and him. I worked methodically, partly entranced by my own purpose there, but the thin, blue partition held nothing back. Words like letters in an alphabet soup and feelings like music at an outdoor concert seemed to waffle up and over the drape. I heard them clearly speaking softly with tenderness. Time seemed to stretch a lifetime to let these lovers chat and muse. I cried quietly during the whole procedure, and never did he move or flinch as if I did not exist poking and pushing. She never looked at me, just him, and her eyes were tearing up, betraying her lighthearted dialogue.

"Babe, don't cry. We can see the movie you want," he offered.

She laughed a little and told him how much she loved him. He told her the same back, and a little hilt in his voice wondered why she was so serious.

"Babe," she exacted, "something has happened, and you are sick and they need to take you to surgery. Babe, it's serious and I love you so much and . . ." Her tears were now tidal waves, and the sobbing grew like a whale moaning under water from the depths of her chest. "I need you to know how much I love you. I need you to know that I will be okay, and you and I will be again one day. Can you say goodbye back to me?" she asked.

I thought God moved her lips and commanded her voice. I thought God was a great puppet master, a great writer of romances, a great lover to love these two and to leave me off to the side, suturing as if I was irrelevant and the catastrophe unreal. What madness to cry into my mask and hope it would absorb every drop before dropping onto my field, tears I could attest were sterile but tainted with empathic pain.

"Babe, it's okay. I know. I heard them talking but I didn't hear them talking. Babe, I love you. Let's see whatever movie you want." He smiled and leaned over a bit to her as I tied my last knot and covered the central line with an adhesive patch. She kissed him, satisfied he understood, but more so happy he did not say goodbye but merely he would be there as planned forever.

Then they said thank yous to each other, maybe to me. It was as if just gratitude blanketed everything, and no one was greedy tugging at it. I took the drape down slowly so as not to startle them, and then suddenly it was time. I mumbled "Thank you" back to everything in the universe and them. The noise flooded in, and a team of people surrounded us all. She and I pushed away from the gurney, and he smiled at only her as he was taken.

The social worker led her away, and I went to clean up. The chief called back over his shoulder, "You get those consents signed?"

"Yeah, I did," I called forward just as he and the team exited the bay, which was still so messy and chaotic. I cleaned up my small contribution to chaos and felt the room meagerly tidier. I sat to chart in the stillness and thought about the awesome events that had unfolded with a kind of acid rising in my gut.

The story goes, the Trauma team successfully operated, and the patient survived hemicorporectomy to leave and enter the ICU. There he caught biological fire with rapid acidosis. Thirty minutes later he was dead, and the day's dust settled on the void where once was a man whose mind lay in the wake of a powerful electrical surge, dreaming only of a movie date with his wife.

♥

Should I

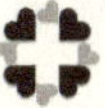

She wrung her hands in the faucet of considerations: Should I or should I not eat protein, drink smoothies, take medicines to lower cholesterol, lose weight, wear compression stockings, stop drinking after 7 p.m., or exercise? At eighty-three years of age, she was an overachiever at heart and took the recommendations she heard to extremes.

"I just worry I'm doing something wrong," she confessed.

Her husband sat beside her, supportive and equally concerned. He gripped his four-pronged cane. His scoliosis set his gaze to my chin, and yet our eyes met as my head tilted in earnest effort to engage the caged soul.

"To be honest, we want to go to Edinburgh to see our grandson graduate with a PhD in History, but we worry we are not healthy enough," she elaborated and he nodded in unison.

I saw no medical concerns and no barriers that would keep the patient from traveling.

"Why wouldn't you be healthy enough?" I inquired, perplexed.

They shifted nervously and she admitted, shyly defeated, "Well, we are old and he is slow and I am fat and his eyes look down a bit and . . ." She trailed and he continued: "I hold people up and I can't stand long and I . . ."

"But our family is literally designing the trip around us," she chimed in.

"And our daughter is orchestrating it all," he prided.

"Honestly," she said, saddened, "he decided yesterday to not go. He told me to go alone."

"I wouldn't hold her back," he puffed gallantly.

"Look at him," she requested. "Do you think he can go?"

He was not my patient. She was my patient, yet I took a look at her husband as if he were once a pedigree stallion being sold for potentially glue, watching him rise and sit and walk. I listened to him talk as I inquired whether he had too much of an ego to use porters and sit in wheelchairs.

"We just went to Michigan and I used a porter the whole way!" he chuckled.

"Not a problem there," she added. "I think his only wound is how he looks down."

"But we have managed to make eye contact the whole time!" I reflected.

He was acknowledged and puffed to be equal in conversation and gaze.

"How can I tell you anything but to go?" I encouraged emphatically, slamming my palm against the table.

The smack was a firecracker, and the two slapped awake like juveniles with sudden funds on their first trip abroad, percolating with anticipation.

"I'm getting so excited now!" she thrilled, and he leaned forward onto his cane.

"So am I now." He laughed and patted her thigh.

"He needed to really hear this," she said, tearing up.

"How can I tell you anything but TO GO?" I repeated, and used my doctorate to push them into embracing a slice of life.

So she set to walk a mile a day till they left to gain stamina, and he set to call the daughter and tell her to book the flights. The smell of Edinburgh in May lingered in the hallways of my office as they pranced away, newlyweds to an idea to be young again. January never seemed so potentiated.

"Oh," by the way, "two days after we return we will have been married sixty years!" she giggled. "We met in second grade!"

He smiled like they had shared every color of crayons already.

"What a tale to share on your anniversary party! Slides of the recent trip abroad?" I teased.

"Wouldn't that be something, Darling." He raised his head to gaze upon her.

Their eyes met, and all the "should I's" were a Red Sea divided to make way for a trip of a lifetime.

♥

Designated Driver

Residency is a mystery to the vast public. It is a constant flip, switch, and climb. Each month the rotation resets and the learning curve starts again in another aspect of the art of medicine. It is an infuriating backslide but sometimes a reprieve. A fresh rotation can help a resident walk away from drudgery or sometimes the reality of too much attachment while still helpless in training.

Gastroenterology rotation: Resident 2nd year, fifth month

She was eighty-seven years old. Her name was Alice. Decades earlier she had a total colectomy. This resulted in dumping syndrome. Every meal dumped out of her within an hour of eating. Methodically timed eating and a diet of 80 percent fiber let her become the designated driver of cronies. She had to drive the group of four to bridge each week. She would poop before she left and when she arrived—and before she left and when she got home. She was the only one with a driver's license, still having keen eyes and fast reflexes.

"I have to renew my license next year," she said.

She came in this time with suddenly uncontrollable diarrhea. It would just run down her leg. She was mentally crisp and thoughtful. I enjoyed speaking with her each morning. My intern, "Little Lucy," and I would joke with her. Lucy was an energetic, bright-eyed, eager girl. She was more than eighteen inches shorter than me. I knew we looked like a circus show to Alice. I endearingly called my intern Little Lucy but she was fierce and quick. Lucy pre-rounded expeditiously and jumped on the task list with the fervor of ascending a mountain before sunset. She nodded when anyone spoke, and I imagine her cogwheels registering, "Got it. Yes. Okay. Done. Got it. Done. Yup. Yes. Got it." She was a resident's dream. "Resident's dream. Got it."

Alice seemed to enjoy fashion and shoes, so we all would lighten the talk of stool output with talk about textures and fabric. She would always ask what we wore under our white coats.

"You two are lovely today!" Alice would say each morning. I think we missed our families and our moms. I think we missed lighthearted bantering and easy speak. Lucy and I would joke with her. I remember even a bright orange scarf Lucy wore. It was the preferred topic one morning. One minute it was about never leaving the hospital, fifteen bowel movements a day, liquid diarrhea described as thick cocoa and then a reprieve, Lucy's orange scarf with a streak of gold, and some squealings of admiration.

Alice's admission became a never-ending failure to firm up her bowel movements. Desperation taught us of an old remedy called tincture of opium. It conjured images of days of opium dens and satin smoke. Creatively, we were going to drug her till she became constipated. She said, "Oh my!"

I wrote the order, flagged the chart, and left for the day.

I arrived the next morning to Alice having less diarrhea but to something worse. Alice had broken her hip during the night. She had gotten up to have a bowel movement and in her opium unsteadiness she slipped on a dripping bit of diarrhea. "Shit," I whispered loudly. "Shit. Got it," Lucy registered, and then I saw her really register it. "Shit. Oh my god. That's horrible. Alice." Lucy awoke out of training, as we all do into the world where we are faced with souls we were training to care for.

Our hearts ached. I was devastated. Our dear Alice. The designated driver of a group of close friends was more broken than when she came in. The feeling of failing laid on me like an elephant, and I could not face Alice. The next step was to have Cardiology clear her for hip surgery. By that afternoon she developed atrial fibrillation. Cardiology deemed her high risk and placed her on digoxin. Orthopedics said they would operate still, not wanting to let a woman die in bed and succumb to pain and the pneumonia of being bedridden.

"Okay. We are back in business. We will do the surgery, fix the diarrhea; she goes back to driving," I checked off loudly on pre-rounds the next morning. Lucy registered the plan, delighted to pivot and continue.

Then the beautiful made-up plan spiraled violently out of control. Alice decided to not have surgery.

The plan was decisive and clear. It made such beautiful sense on paper. Digoxin, surgery, diarrhea controlled, rehab, home driving. What was the problem? Digoxin, surgery, diarrhea controlled, rehab, home driving!

We went in to talk to Alice and beg her. Alice held my hand and I cried openly, uncontrollably. Lucy stood just behind me.

"Please, Alice," I begged. I was reduced to begging. I had never begged a patient before, but we were supposed to fix her and get her back to her duties. People needed her. She had the only license. Were physicians supposed to beg patients?

"No, it's okay. I know you both want me to have surgery but it's okay. I know it's time. It's just too much now," Alice said, reassuring me. Alice was doctoring us. We needed reassurance. We needed Alice to teach us how to stop even if on paper it looked perfect. The weight of the white coat could not hide our disappointment. Lucy and I begged her over and over. Alice never wavered and looked at peace.

Alice needed to rest, so we left the room and I collapsed in a chair. Lucy looked at me and I am sure had no idea what to think of an upper-level resident so destroyed. Over and over I thought, "A beautiful soul will leave having died from slipping on diarrhea."

Lucy nodded slowly as she patted and stroked my back. "We got too close, I think," Lucy surmised.

I cried typing up the note. I cried while eating. I cried driving home. Alice lulled off into a morphine haze, happy to not have a bowel movement ruin her peace. Her heart slowed and over the day she faded.

Never does the story leave me. I can only hope patients sense my carefulness but also my strong desire to get them back to their lives. "Be patient," I say. "Be strong," I say. I still beg a lot. "Please. Please try," I plead. Above all this, I hope patients sense I respect their choice and narrative.

God, help us not die a humiliating death after spinning out of control on a patch of filth. God, help us choose bravely staying or exiting life. God, help us to execute the patient's storyline despite the pain and longing in our hearts for easy choices that are not there to be had.

♥

The Story of Eight Kidneys

Cindy is my contemporary. While we were in high school, I was somewhere fighting to stay awake and to get ahead and Cindy was somewhere fighting to survive.

Go, go, GO. I was thinking of nothing more than being a doctor. I never knew that I would be Cindy's doctor one day.

She was born with blocked kidneys, and every time she peed, urine shot up into them and gave her pain. While she was just a kid, her two kidneys failed.

Her mom blamed herself because Cindy suffered. She donated her kidney. While I read and studied, pouring my hours into books and feeling determined to milk the universe, Cindy had starts and sputters. At times she tasted normal life. She tried to believe it was going to be better, but being young you can't see straight even when straight exists.

By 1992, I graduated high school and marched with scholarship in hand. Simultaneously, Cindy faced the failure of her transplant, and again her mom blamed herself.

Over the next four years, I fought to get noticed, to achieve the seemingly unattainable medical school admission. I joked that to achieve my dream I "would sell my kidney" while Cindy somewhere "would buy it" being of not so humorous a notion to need it.

By 2006, my dreams were all true and Cindy was still on dialysis, still dreaming. She had been living on dialysis for almost fifteen years.

Unknown to me, Cindy had been my partner's patient while I studied and trained for those fifteen years. I chanced to become her nephrologist being both in our thirties. Newly married to a man who would come and scratch her back as she dialyzed, Cindy began her journey with me.

She for years declined another transplant, having grown weary. We all accepted her choice, sad to think of youth on a timer. Thankfully, my partner convinced her, and she easily listed as she was otherwise very healthy and we waited.

By 2009 she was transplanted for the second time and began another insane journey with starts and sputters. She remained with another physician for the first two years post-transplant. She dared then to live and make up time all the while feeling she was on borrowed time again. She sorted her restlessness and dared to dream of starting a family and having babies. The first attempts were hard, and when she was finally pregnant she lost the baby in August 2011. I made partner that same year in my practice while Cindy fought for the common joys of motherhood. The antirejection medications that kept her off dialysis also made conception challenging.

By 2011, Cindy returned to me. I was busy building a practice and holding a thousand lives like a ferris wheel ride. By the time we reengaged, I was seasoned and sure of everything as much as she was unsure if she was really stable and remotely human.

One day we tackled an infection, but before we decided on any antibiotics Cindy took a pregnancy test and, well, she tested positive! That began the next nine months of swollen anticipation. Soon we learned she was to have twins!

I watched her tiny body that never grew above that of a tween due to her child years battling kidney disease triple! How she held those babies I have no idea! We counted our blessings and the kidneys she held, one transplanted and four in the lives inside her and historically two she was born with and one her mother gave her that had failed. These eight kidneys stacked and paved a passage towards the daunting pinnacle of motherhood.

Her expanding uterus was squishing the kidney transplant, threatening again obstruction, and we began to count days like sand grains, hoping we collected enough for a castle in the sky. At thirty-three weeks and six days, we threw her in the hospital to monitor and prepare her and those babies for delivery. When the babies came, she knew suddenly why her own mom had worried and worried.

This is the tale of eight kidneys, now three lives. This is the tale of my friend and contemporary who at thirty-seven has lived with endurance a race like no other. This is modern medicine meets maternal instincts. This is why medicine fights to find solutions that make the life force unstoppable.

♥

The Piece of Pie

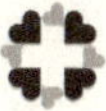

My partner retired.

We divided his patient panel like a warm pie. I inherited a slice as a very special patient. He had received his wife's kidney a decade earlier, and he was a quiet and capable man. He had a mustache like a Conquistador. What made him special was his ease and gratitude.

The years passed uneventfully and then he got COVID at the height of the delta variant.

I met his wife near the elevator in the hospital just as his oxygen requirement increased to near unsustainable levels. She was frantic and we chatted. I recall I grabbed her shoulders to tell her to brace herself should things spiral.

Remarkably, he survived brilliantly! But the next year was a complete cluster of coronary issues with pulmonary congestion and fatigue. He never complained. In fact, I needed to teach him to voice his needs, less he got discharged each time without even a wheelchair escort or a wave.

One day while I was in a Walgreens parking lot doing my own errands, his wife called the office frantic, as was her custom late in the week, late in the day, every week. I returned the call despite my day off. They needed to commit to a second heart catheterization, then maybe a valve replacement, but even with all of that he could crash into renal failure.

"All in," I declared and told them life has many challenges so one must have also guts to face them. "Living is taking risks." I thrusted his chips forward.

"All in," she agreed, and he burped up a "Yup" to settle.

The cardiologist was a prince; caring, concerned, considerate. He called me twice, speaking at length and with metered reservations but also with a kind of courage that his training and experience afforded him. I thanked him for his courtesy to call and the collegial way he approached collaborative care.

We did Phase 1. He returned to the office stable but breathless. We began to plan Phase 2.

Less than a week later another frantic call, where he could barely speak. His wife urged him go to the hospital. He only said, "Nope."

"Talk some sense into him," she begged me.

I reviewed his prior hospitalization and guessed at a workup and projected the possibility of pushing for an urgent valve replacement.

"Nope," he huffed. Slowly he squeezed out, "They have worked and worked . . . on this . . . and they don't have much to do that's . . . easy and I'm . . . just tired of it . . . all."

His wife let out a visceral scream. She yelled at him loudly, "You are going to die! You are going to die right here in front of me!"

The screaming was so loud that it punched though the receiver and into my office. My assistant came in wondering if I was okay or assaulted.

"Sir, there are three things here," I said, dividing the perspective. "How you are feeling, how your wife is feeling, and what if anything hard or easy we can hope to do. Will you go to the hospital and let us try, or are you tired and ready?"

He paused, and I imagine he looked over at his wife with the heavy, thoughtful eyes I had seen before.

"I'm not going," he announced. I heard him walk away from the phone gently and slowly. I imagined one of two matching armchairs he headed toward, resolved to sit and not argue about how to live his life or die his death to satisfy others

His wife and I allowed his choice, heavy with thoughts and hopeful he might on his own reconsider.

We hung up, and the next day I got a call. He had died in his sleep peacefully. The messenger left a number "should I want to call." I could not imagine a different choice.

"Hello?" she answered. Her frantic and recently screaming tone had deflated so much that I hardly recognized her voice.

"Hello, it's Dr. Robey," I offered. As if a stage properly set for production, I drew the curtain back and asked kindly, "Tell me everything that happened."

She inhaled and then told a tale of how she had hung up and realized immediately she just needed to support him. They sat together and then had dinner. She drifted off to sleep despite trying to stay up to see if he needed anything. She surmised he had sat up and got a piece of pie and some cookies, as she found crumbs and a blueberry-stained plate the next day. She recalled at some point that he had returned to bed, for she had grown accustomed to placing a hand on his chest to feel him breathing and felt her hand naturally find the rhythm of his breaths . . . or perhaps she had dreamt it after so many nights doing it and had declared it so.

Nevertheless, she awoke by 2 a.m. to the absence of expectations of a rising chest.

"I knew right away when he died," she attested. "The stillness of his chest woke me, and I did CPR right away, but he was gone," she explained.

Suddenly, I was her husband. Pain seared up my foot and leg into my chest, and I heard the fork clang against the ceramic beige plate with a green and maroon rim, but I ignored it groaning a crumb out my mouth. I tasted still blueberries as I chewed a thoughtful peanut butter cookie, letting crumbs fall wherever they willed. I wanted nothing more, and then I readied myself for bed and climbed in next to my wife to one last time place her donated left kidney in my right pelvis to her left side properly; a pair for a pair.

Being him briefly, I was home and then I was in heaven, and I could not tell that I left anything behind for I was free and breathing easily at last.

Returning back to myself on the phone with the wife's soft sobs, I felt the odd flatness of my office. As we chatted more about the years past and hurdles surmounted, I wondered if I opened my office door I would find the hallway recoiled back to only three dimensions divorced of empathy.

"I guess in ways we have been readied since he had COVID and all the chaos that time threatened us with. I guess in ways we had to accept it to let it lay the way it would today," I surmised.

His wife was satisfied and grateful. She was tired and sad but at peace. It was such a force of effort to constantly work the problems her husband faced, but it spent every last ounce of her self-doubt and thus freed her completely.

"I did the best I could all these years. After we hung up last, I just looked at him in the corner of the living room so determined to quit while ahead and I had to stop and just let it be," she confessed.

"We didn't leave anything on the table," I agreed.

"I had to give him dignity and it cost me everything, but it was worth it," she swore.

I told her she was extraordinary and that dignity is a pricey thing indeed but of great, immeasurable value. I thanked them both for the opportunity to know firsthand two universes so exquisitely complete and unique but masterful together.

She thanked me for my time, which I imagine over the years totaled some twenty-odd hours. I felt that was a minimal cost indeed for knowledge like I had acquired of human strength, endurance, and support. All this effort, for transplantation, for diabetes, for renal disease, for COVID, for heart disease . . . and in the end for love, was me running into them over and over till his time came. There is no fast valor, no more attainable thing for a human to do in God's image but to lay down a sword and command an end coming or to rest a hand on a loved one's chest till it rises no more and choose to rise ourselves against the weight of the grief of losing our better half.

♥

The Autopsy

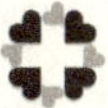

They say the dead speak more than the living. Maybe because they have no choice but to be immediately naked before the questionings.

The walls, white with subway tiles, pushed back the light and noise. The room—sparse except for the door we walked in through, the uniformed stainless steel, rectangular tables, the loud air vents demarcating each station, the hoses that hung from the ceiling, and the water that sloshed about the drains—was an icebox of frozen misery. I entered to the sound of echoes and water being sprayed. It seemed a fish market, not by smell but by rhythm and noises. The dampness and cold like a morning dock coming alive invited four teams. Each team had a pathologist and a rising resident. There were, however, thirteen people in the room, four of whom no longer had much to say—or so I thought. I was to be the guest that day to stories, a speechless and shivering medical student.

"Here, put on these," the resident said, handing me long shoe covers. They provided some warmth while they hugged against my flimsy scrubs. The floors around the drains were pooling water, and the dampness made me uneasy. Such a place needed knee-high galoshes. The pathologists all wore the heavier armor. Everyone weakly protected their hearts.

The main metal table in the far back was the one for the hour. We walked through the room to it. I cringed as I approached. Upon the far table was a small, naked girl. She had bruises all over and a cut above her left eyebrow slightly covered by a locket of muddy hair. There appeared to be a depression on the left temporal. When her blond hair was brushed away, a large bruise necklaced her throat. She was thin but not terribly so. She lay pale and exposed. Naked in so many ways, she had no befitting protection or warmth on the metal table in the sterile room. She was alone among strangers. Who would hold her hand and love her across the busy street of investigations? Her eyes were closed. I imagined them blue as the file reported.

She should have been in a soft room with curtains and fuzzy purple pillows or on a lap of her mother, giggling and shy upon our approach. Her lips were visibly blue-tinged, and she just lay there devoid of childish things. I instantly felt sick to see her little, lifeless body. It was altogether a wild stew of emotions to see a dead child. I felt my entire worth tested against her limited mortality, a fraction of what I selfishly took for granted in my quadrupled years beyond her status. I was never going to be a dead child on a table. So, there she lay as proof that children die and proof still of the wicked things that kill them.

"I always secure their eyelids," the resident said, tapping them gently closed so they would not peek open to criticize our touch, which was already too rough.

I closed my own eyes for a minute, and the child's image stayed. What was the last thing she saw?

I watched the autopsy, listening to the analysis. I tried to focus on the anatomy and technique. The entire room and the noise that echoed became the naked child's outline. I could not see past that one detail. I noticed the pathologist sniffling and her mask growing foggy. She was crying softly.

"I learn the story in pieces. First on paper, then by a timeline of bruises and a growing list of injuries," she shared. "I cry my way through, and it pains me to know they can't speak at all for themselves."

I had to leave just thirty-five minutes into the autopsy. It was all too much for my constitution, and I felt my legs detaching from under me. I was too naïve in life and in evil to bear much on my first day.

Later when the team finished, they found me quiet in the ready room.

"Do you have to do autopsies on children?" I asked as I considered my courage to be a pathologist. The slides and gross specimens partitioned out—all linked to people with lives and hopes—seemed daunting to learn and place in context, but the understanding of death and the method of dying seemed an art I could not remove myself personally far enough from.

"You have to serve everyone." The pathologist laid her soul on the table to show the unique organ she had. "Especially when no one served them in life."

♥

Your Face

The daughter called me at 9:30 p.m.

"My dad died tonight but he's okay now. He's talking and stuff. Anyway, we need a current medication list," she opened.

I was a bit confused, though open to the casual possibility he was "okay now."

He had been at a restaurant with family and suddenly fell forward into his steak, evoking his defibrillator to fire three times. Paramedics came before anyone around them got dessert and revived him fully with a series of strong chest compressions. Then, he arrived at the hospital "okay now."

I found him in his room with the covers pulled to his chin like an oversized boy in a foreign bed. He looked at me flatly. I spoke. He stared.

The next day they rolled him to the CATH lab and threaded his highways and freeways. Behind their masks they furrowed and frowned. He stared. They whispered to each other and talked increasingly loudly to him. "You. Have. Major. Blockages!" they informed. He stared. They repeated themselves. He stared. They gave up having informed him and charting they did.

I came into his room after he had returned, and they coordinated a heave to return him to his bed. They seemed overly extended with pleasantries, the way people are when they feel awkward. I talked to him with all the animation of Disney about the ramifications of bypass surgery on moderately impaired kidneys. He stared.

When I was leaving, I turned to him and shared, "One more thing because I have known you for years and can read your face the best, and still I admittedly find myself searching for clues that you understand what I'm saying. Be sure you tell them you have Parkinson's flat affect so they don't fall victim to over-explaining, over-expressing their point, or under-estimating you."

He stared.

Then he smiled slyly and affirmed, "I got you. Thanks for knowing me."

♥

Code Status

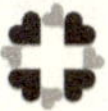

Sometime ago, maybe five years ago, she would take him to dialysis. Everyone said he was the nicest, most pleasant man. He never complained about the chore of attending three times a week. In time he was a star student, though quietly he forgot frivolous details, most new names, and the seemingly barrage of various recommendations given daily. The transplant team was impressed by his overall success and found nothing alarming, so he was quickly listed.

A short time later a perfect match led to a fated twist. He awoke from the anesthesia after his kidney transplant oddly and gravely forgetful. Dementia seeped into the gyrus like gravy, and he drooled a little when he started to fall asleep in a chair.

His new kidney transplant was a beauty, and the days of dialysis faded away to a working kidney transplant but also a future instead in a wheelchair, constantly unable to hold a thought.

Somehow his wife knew his every gesture. She hired a caregiver who grew to understand he liked baseball and Mars bars.

Eventually the wife was free to live a life, and sometimes she would go to the casino or out with friends. Eventually she slept with the caregivers, being lonely and in an awkward position. She would never leave her husband. There were no winners or losers, just compromises, and no one could say clearly why he had returned a vacant man after what should have been a freeing surgery.

"Just seems a rare reaction to anesthesia. Not a stroke," the trusted transplant doctor explained. Ironically, that trusted doctor died suddenly in his sleep one day, and so he was surpassed by a seemingly sicker soul. The transplanted man had multiple admission for grave sepsis and yet survived.

One day, for example, they had noticed he was not awake for a baseball game and would not take the favorite candy bar. Oddly, the drooling stopped, and he was less of a mess. "Well, dry all over," his wife considered. He was watered and fed through a tube inserted down his nose, and he returned each day to once again become the man in the chair the wife and caregivers swore watched baseball and craved Mars bars and drooled, being better hydrated.

Every admission on the precipice of death, the care team would discuss his code status.

"You know he will not regain his mental faculties. You know he may in fact die this time," they would say.

But she insisted he remain a Full Code.

"Why do they always exhaust me with such negative talk?" the wife asked me. "Why do they give up?" she accused.

It seemed a manner of perspective, one she could not possibly fully weigh while living in a bubble of evolved adult disability.

"He has become significantly disabled, but only you can easily see the person behind the eyes when open," I justified.

She acquiesced to see the other side of a ravine, and yet no one met her remotely on her side of that unknowable chasm where she saw her husband and we all saw a shell. She ceded his setbacks, but no one truly would credit his personhood to her appreciation. One day he died in a storm like none before, and her shoulders slumped. She was tired and simultaneously freed, and she thanked everyone for trying. As she left the hospital, she tried once more to humanize her husband.

"You know he used to play baseball. I think when he watched it he came alive like no other time, and I wish you all could have seen that just once," she scolded and left the hospital unapologetic about his right to personhood. There was a brief moment of silence as we contemplated our shame, and then the noises started back up again to ease our difficulty accepting our own fragility and ephemeral mark.

♥

Fields Before Us

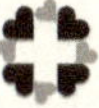

He was one of the youngest patients I had. He never said much. He tried to look me in the eyes but it was hard. I looked down and away so he could look up and speak up. Everything about renal failure intimidated him, and though he spoke firmly it would be easy to crush him and fill him with dread and doubt. He refused a fistula in his arm because he was a musician and wrote songs and "needed to play the guitar." When he said "needed," there was pain and longing in his voice like a country song itself.

"Possibly numb fingers" after fistula access surgery meant he could not strum the chords he heard in his heart. Also, it would "kill my soul, ma'am," he swore. I let it go because a man's soul is nothing to put on the line month after month. He said no to a kidney transplant referral too. His two brothers had offered to donate a kidney, but he declined quietly, not wanting to be a burden. I let go asking about a fistula as he held on thinly, but every month for three years I asked about kidney transplantation considerations. He always said, "No, I'm fine, ma'am."

"He was special, my boy," his father choked up. "He would tell me about dialysis and about the blind girl he sat next to and how sorry he was she was there suffering and how she shouldn't be there," his father shared.

I never fully know what my patients observe in the common treatment room or how it moves them inside like fire burning for all time.

Extraordinary is a man tethered to a machine himself yet only sees that another person should not be there.

He had three kids. Called his first girl "gorgeous." The twins were born during his first year on dialysis. The story goes when the twins became older and climbed every day on his lap and his first gorgeous girl started school, well, he needed more life, he needed more time. He would cut his dialysis treatments short to get that precious time to pick up his girl at the corner each day. I let it be because those five to fifteen minutes meant he had love waiting around a corner. It made the other three hours and forty-five minutes of his treatment endurable. I was never a stickler. I was never one to insist he miss the duty of meeting his daughter to walk her home to make perfect his numbers.

"Okay, so you know the drill. I have to ask if you would like me to refer you for transplantation," I asked again, as always.

At the corner outside a school emptying out, a gorgeous little girl waited for her daddy to arrive and sing her a song he had written while driving. He would sing how golden her hair was and why rivers should smile if ever her bare feet "slip on into cool waters carefree." Those notes lingered in the air for days till I saw him on a routine visit and he sang to me, "Yes, I do want you to refer me for transplant." He rewrote his tune and my heart fluttered like a butterfly around a flower.

"Yes!" I exclaimed in a subdominant major.

And then the story continued. After a successful transplant, he left my circle for some time on the motor of a new kidney.

Two years later I found him in the hospital with some nausea, unable to hold down important antirejection medicines. Within a night he was righted, and I reminded him to follow up with me or the transplant center if he was still in their line of sight. "No, actually they said they wanted me to start coming back to you," he beamed, so we made a date to reconvene.

He arrived in the midst of the COVID pandemic as a telemedicine visit. We recapped all the twists and turns and ran the labs and medication list, and he made his next appointment outside the projected lines of changed days. I promised him in three months we would certainly be safe to meet in person. "I'm sure by then society will know more and we will be sorted." I hung up on that last line.

Four weeks later I got notice to sign a death certificate. He had been found dead and I was his listed physician. Being under the care of any physician made his death "of natural causes," and the thirteen medical examiners in the state were so busy with COVID cases that despite my begging for an autopsy they closed the case. A few phone calls later I found that a private autopsy cost $3,000. The family thanked me for the information but the need to know why Daniel had died soon diminished under the grief of losing him, the outrageous cost to find out, and the compounded grief of no proper funeral given social distancing. The crush of COVID left so many unburied and unsung.

"Doc," his father asked, "do you . . . My wife wants to know if you . . . well, did he ever tell you if he wanted to be buried or cremated?"

Long ago, Daniel and I spoke of Tennessee. Apparently, it is a songwriter's dream to be there in the heartland of music. I had let Daniel settle imperfectly on so many medical matters, sensing little mattered so much to change a man's soul by force. I listened to his melody instead and only asked those things he could not fail to do. This gentle and acceptable lenience allowed me to know something about Daniel. Long ago, Daniel told me that being in Tennessee was just all the joys of life before his kids. After his kids, he had another heartland—being near them—and that deep affection overcame his fears and enabled him to fight so he could be present. Daniel was a passionate split soul who refused to give death a note, his melody driven by love of music and family.

"I'm not sure, sir, but I would guess he would want cremation and his ashes spread, some in Tennessee, to finally be in two places with all the abilities to do what he wanted as if things had not changed because of kidney failure or death," I offered.

"Yes, that sounds right, Doc. I thank you. He did love Tennessee as much as he loved those kids of his," he was reminded.

I do not know why Daniel died. There were no signs of criminality, save the unsatisfying verdict of "cardiac arrest" or "end stage renal failure" I was left to write on his death certificate to release his body. Lyrics floated up to him on forever-tuned guitar strings to tell him I was very sad to see his untimely passing in a field before me.

Fields Before Us

She was prettier than the sky
Set apart from city life
Brought me joy before I die
Fields alive with wildflowers
Kids climbing on me
Suddenly
I needed to stretch out time
I needed to find a way besides

I don't know where this road goes
I don't know all the notes to sing
Bring me back to Tennessee where I belong
I am so far from simple things
On the shores of self-harm thinking of
All the things weighing on me

They say I could choose
But all I saw was you
Waiting at the corner

Fields Before Us

She was prettier than the sky
Set apart from city life
I don't know where this road goes
I don't know all the notes to sing
Bring me back to Tennessee where I belong

They say I could choose
But all I saw was you
Waiting at the corner
Waiting at the corner
Waiting at the corner of the fields before us

♥

Nate

The morning crisped to our walk down the hallway. My geriatric fellow in tow, I knocked and entered rooms and lives up and down the hallway. My fellow was fresh on the scene and had the soul of compassion already. Today would be a treat for us.

Room 324D

Three days ago Mr. Salvatore was admitted, extremely short of breath.

"I thought I would die," he reflected after.

Truly he would have with an oxygen saturation of 72 percent if unattended.

After days of diuresis and steroids, he sat in his bed, propped up with the right arm slung over the right railing and the left arm unusually arched, resting on the pillow.

He spoke with a boom, and despite me meeting him for the first time that morning he commanded some advantage. He was seen by my partner and he corrected my pronunciation of my partner's name. I was not put off but logged the posture as evidence of likely a high military background and some medical knowledge. It turned out as we spoke and I inquired that he was indeed retired military, and his son was an accomplished physician, the head of a pediatric department.

We mapped out our plan and purpose and his delicate balance between cardiac and pulmonary mayhem against chronic kidney disease. His smaller-framed and apologetic wife stood by.

"I must ask because I have got to get this out," she interrupted as if learned from years of holding her voice. "How exactly are his kidneys, because once before he was so sick he almost needed dialysis."

I explained his current status and the room relaxed, reassured that though dynamic and in flex there was room to yield and accommodate the needs of his heart and lungs. His wife thanked me. He nodded approval. I backed up and pivoted to exit the room, ending up at the foot of the bed where I could see Mr. Salvatore straight on. Again I was struck by how his left arm laid as an arch across the pillow.

He spoke, so I stopped and stood.

"You know, I have been thinking a lot about my grandson, Nate." He flung the non sequitur into the space between us.

I felt the geriatric fellow shift into a sigh as we were going someplace long and unnecessary. What did Nate have to do with hypoxia and kidney failure? Accustomed to strange twists, I just waited to see why we were venturing randomly to places seemingly irrelevant.

Nate was a lovely and intelligent boy. "He was my everything. You never met a better boy. He would lay right on my chest under my left arm, in my armpit even, and rest his head to watch TV with me. I even asked him once why he would choose the left side. He said because it smelled better than the right armpit!" Mr. Salvatore bellowed. His wife laughed at the memory and touched her husband's leg. Tears welled up in her eyes.

Three years ago, at ten years of age, Nate died in a tragic accident when a tractor tipped over and crushed him. He didn't die instantly. The weight of the tractor suffocated him and his other grandmother, unable to lift the tractor up, watched the life drain from him. The tractor laid on Nate for some time till it could be lifted. The limp body was vacant of the lovely soul that loved life so vigorously and sweetly.

I stood paralyzed by the details and story. I did not understand why I should be in the room a little too long to land into this horrible image and knowledge.

"You know," Mr. Salvatore started as if out of a daze and back into the now, "I'm the kind of guy that leaves as soon as I get better. I usually hurry out and fight staying."

The room came into focus. The position of Mr. Salvatore, his wife to the right by his bedside standing, the geriatric fellow quietly standing just behind me to the right, me standing at the foot of the bed looking dead straight with Mr. Salvatore, and . . . Nate resting in that otherwise oddly placed left arm arch all bloomed in a perfect 3D puzzle.

"Mr. Salvatore," I chilled, "you have gifted us with Nate, and for all the world I wish I could give you him right now from where I stand. But I can show you something if you bear with me this time. You usually leave too soon, but you agree to stay this time to allow me to titrate properly your diuretics and rebalance you. You usually resist but this time you don't feel inclined to," I summarized. He nodded, agreeable. "Sir, you have been sitting with your left arm arched out as if holding Nate there, and I swear he is here with you and coaxing you to relax and stay and be well. Nate loves you."

The whole room bowed. Stunned by reality, we felt humbled. It was a definite moment of perfect arrangement, and I knew it was real because Mr. Salvatore gasped and tears exploded forth.

"Yes! Yes. That's what thinking of Nate for days now has done. Yes. I feel him here and I didn't want to leave," he exclaimed. He looked down at his chest, and the muscles in his left arm twitched. I thought about how I cradle my own children and the inedible impression they leave in that space against my bosom.

The weight of love spun us all. We thanked each other for the moment. We had to part to breathe, and when the geriatric fellow and I left we walked in silence.

"In every day and every week you chance to stop and find the beauty in what you do," I broke, speaking to the fellow. "Be sure to find love in the incredible lives of patients and witness it as their doctor and reflect it back to them. It will keep you in love with what you do and why."

♥

Dear Alice

Dear Alice,

I went into see Dr. Robey today. You remember Dr. Robey. She's the tall one, the one with the shoes you always like. Remember how we were going to Costco and before we did we stopped by her office for my appointment and she hugged you because it had been so long since you'd been in with me? I don't figure you do but maybe since you hugged her back and smiled brighter than I had seen you smile you remembered her and that day. You said you remembered her when she hugged you that day and, boy, I was happy at Costco walking around hearing you say you remembered her.

I went in today. I would go every month if I could! She's always greeting me like she misses me and looking worried like you did if my shirt isn't tucked right or I'm skinny-looking. Today she said I had filled back out and that I looked a good weight. I told her I could gain no more back because of the suit! Remember that suit? I told her how back forty years we were going to that high school reunion and you found that western suit at that shoe soling store. Remember? You had wandered off while I squared away soling my boots and you found that suit. Ha! I wandered, looking for you, calling out your name while looking like I was a lost kid. I finally found you looking over that suit, and you were so fixated on getting that suit for $200! I can't believe how long it took me to get you out of the store and home. Oh, we fought about that suit. I was just going to get a shirt and some slacks for $40 tops but you kept going on and on. I said, "I love you, honey, but that's crazy."

Next morning do you remember how you woke up, made a fine breakfast, then got dressed? I said, "Where are you going?" and you said so certain, "*We* are going to get that suit!"

I told Dr. Robey about that moment. She laughed because I guess she was thinking how little you were next to me and me going to get my keys to drive you back to the store to have your way. Well, I told her I only wore that suit once and then forgot about it. I told her I went through my closet last week and found it way in the back! I was pushing back a shirt and found it! I thought it was so crazy to think on that day you found the suit in the store and how we fought over it. Well, I tried it on. It fits! And I told Dr. Robey I can't be gaining no weight! I can't believe it fit.

I told Dr. Robey I'm going to wear it to your services and how I wish you could see me in it. You know what she said? Alice, she said you had seen me in it. That the vision and memory were so concretely made forty years ago that you wouldn't ever forget, and I just was so happy my heart nearly exploded. I just want you to remember how much I love you and see me again like that guy you wanted to show off in a $200 suit. You will remember, right? Dr. Robey says you were so very certain about this suit that there's no way you'd forget it.

I miss you, Alice. I do. Come see me in this suit you picked out. I'll be wearing it for you. I would do anything for you.

Love,
Jacob

♥

This Place

Hello darlings

This place
Heaven's gates are opening for you
And the loud noise you heard was just its latch
Shhhhhh
"We never oil the hinges or spare the lock. The keying and swinging wakes the Angels to come greet you."
I know you are soothed by my smell and my presence
They burn incense here
That catches the breezes and ride the sunshine as family gets together and
Those are pillows filled with sleepy time
Those are candy treats
Those are dolls and trucks and toys
I know you are aware that part of my spirit has been sent forth in casual flip-flops
And laughter
I will see you fully soon
Silly bugs
Sweet loves
For time is a wrinkle and fold

I hold you both in my deepest heart
And though I stay here
Just a little while
The Angels will make sure to clothe you in my arms
And have ready seemingly my eyes only for your smiles and seemingly
my ears only for your whispers
Heaven is all these great things all at once
Your joys and comforts come to best each moment
Dress content with amusement
And soon, soon enough I will be there so you can tell me all about it
"Oh mama, there was this one time . . ."
I love you
Remember clearly my womb and my pride
You came from this place of wonderment
And so, for now you return inside my dreams and hopes
I will find you both in time
Till then I have sent forth part of my very grace
To accompany you both
Sweet passage
To this place

♥

The Opioid Crisis

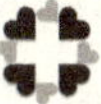

He walked out of the fields of Iowa, mending a fence in the back part of eight acres, and into my office with his third wife. His first wife was a real tyrant and a nag. His second wife was the love of his life, but pancreatic cancer ravaged her. After their ten short years of idyllic marriage, she was gone just months after the diagnosis.

"I can't live alone, Mary," he told his sister after.

Within seven months of his second wife's passing, he married his third wife. They traveled, and she diligently managed all the affairs. He clung desperately to her brilliance and doted on her. They would fight often because she tired of taking charge of their lives. Unfortunately, he never rose fully to meet her growing fatigue.

In 2012 he was extremely exhausted and "ached all over." He required pain medication to help "have energy to mend the fences." A roundabout workup found a Stage 3 A renal cell cancer that invaded the main vein of his body. He successfully had the cancer removed but remained victim to waves of fatigue. The B symptoms made recurrence an ever worry.

He arrived at my office cancer-free but still hooked on pain medications in quarter tablets to get through a day. We addressed addiction and scaling back pain medications. We discussed depression and anxiety. He said he tried my suggestions but still found himself using narcotics intermittently to "get to mending the fences" and nearly begged for them.

He could never pinpoint the pain. Mending fences sounded hard, and he sounded high doing it. I could never exact the right and wrong but scaled the quantity to some thirty tablets every three months, which he then fractioned.

Eventually his third wife left him. In all honesty, I was surprised given that at office visits she seemed very devoted and cordial.

"They fought one day in 2014 and she said, 'In two years I will leave you,'" his sister Mary later shared. "I begged him to get his things in order, which he managed to do a little but never well. Marcy just took care of so much, and he just didn't even know how to manage a bank deposit. In the end, she took everything he had."

In 2016, he arrived at my office without a wife.

"She left me, Doc," he began. He seemed to have processed the bulk of the reality before arriving. We talked about this new fate, and he reconciled to stand again. I commended him. I supported him. Unfortunately, under increasing pressure to continue reducing and exiting chronic narcotics prescribing, I had to inform him during that same visit that I would begin cutting back prescriptions of narcotics to not prescribe. We talked again about addiction and symptoms of withdrawal as well as a possible psychiatric or pain specialist referral. He had managed to reduce to minimal usage but clung to them, unsure how to battle vague pain. Also, there was a new pain in his left rib that caught him at every breath. However, his remaining kidney was on the right.

He took the news in stride, and we focused on ruling out recurrent cancer-causing pain on the left lower flank. He had images done that honed in on a piece of metal wire that had been part of his prior left nephrectomy that appeared dislodged. We searched for several surgeons and one finally agreed to remove the foreign body that November.

"He bought this gun at a gun show in October," Mary overlapped later with a detail.

Immediately after the surgery he was significantly better and was not using any narcotics most days. Twenty pills would last him nearly six months.

I saw him last in February 2017. He was mending fences now in another small town, trying to build a life alone. He thanked me for helping him find a surgeon. I reluctantly wrote the prescription for twenty tablets of pain medication to use for pain. My dilemma was with kidney disease, one kidney, and an inability to use common pain relievers, he needed something for pain after long days working outside. What was I going to do to end the opioid crisis, and what would the day look like when I would no longer provide him any route for pain relief?

I put my head down as my last gesture to him, deep in thought about how to manage his pain as well as my prescribing responsibilities and the nation's opioid crisis. The weight of failure and my directness for challenging a poorly supported social problem exhausted me till I pushed it away to enter another room. I did not look him in the eye that day as we parted. I hurried on, shaking the unclear burden off me, for I had no answers that felt right. Months later I would learn more about inadequacies to address the opioid crisis.

"Hello?" she answered.

"Hello, Mary?" I addressed. "It's Dr. Robey. I got a message you called about your brother while I was away."

"Oh yes, thank you for calling," she introduced herself. "We have never met, but I did come to your office once with Ted. He made me wait in the waiting room, but I have heard only great things. Ted really appreciated you and your help."

"Mary, what happened?" I pressed.

A sibling void opened like a black hole being born.

"Well, Dr. Robey," she inhaled slowly, then exhaled. "Ted rigged a gun he bought and shot himself. I call every week and if I don't get him, he usually calls back. But this last time he didn't, and I got worried and sent someone to find him and . . ." She began to sob. "He must've been dead five days," she surmised.

I saw myself months prior walking out of the exam room with him following, but some part of me was deep in thought then, obscuring the other part of me that would have looked at Ted rising to walk out behind me and maybe had seen something telling or would have taken his hand and shaken goodbye. I saw the two me's thinking about a problem more than the person, and I hated that equation drawn 70/30. I should have looked in his eyes that last time. I had seen him fumble with the prescription I handed him. I perhaps had seen something that I rushed away from. My mind reeled. Maybe if I had looked at him it would have anchored him. Maybe if I had touched him as we parted it would have anchored him.

Why? Why did he do this when he never missed an appointment? He had told me every intimate detail, and like a priest I had heard his confessions. We had fought to find a surgeon to cut his flesh. We had cured a pain jabbing his left side with every breath. He had survived cancer. He had survived loss. He had mended fences, and we would have figured out how to keep on.

Mary recounted details that meant Ted was walking both right and left. While seeking surgery, he had bought a gun. While speaking of moving on, he had felt only miserably alone.

"He never got over Sally, his second wife, dying. Marcy was good to him, but I think she got tired of him being sick. She wanted to travel, and he couldn't keep up," Mary shared. "He kept saying this last year that if only he didn't get sick Marcy would not have left and how he didn't want to be alone."

My heart broke. The pieces blew out into the wheat fields of Iowa and got lost past a part of a fence never mended. Ted felt alone, and mending fences felt like solving some part of that.

"He told everyone it was just you and me he trusted," Mary damned me.

"Oh, Mary," I sobbed. "I'm so sorry. I never saw it coming like this. He never spoke of suicide. He fought each visit to feel better. We won many times. He had plans and goals. We reviewed them and he made honest progress. I didn't see this."

I could hear Mary nodding.

Mary had recognized her brother's grief and loneliness and offered him visits and company. Early on she offered him addiction counseling.

"Oh, Mary! For the last years I have been slowly weaning his narcotics but offering alternatives and referrals. Do you think he grew desperate?" I pained to realize. The opioid crisis laid at my doorstep like a volcanic eruption of flesh blown about as a bullet entered a man's head.

"I don't know. I called every week. He seemed so much better after that surgery to take out that metal thing," she replied deep in disorientation. "I don't know," she sobbed.

We spoke and cried for a long while.

"Mary, I don't know what is going on," I offered. "I guess I do know we are the last standing and stand for each other. Without the other we might be more confused. I guess I want to believe Ted left us each other, and I can only assure you that I didn't see it. You know he would've told me. I didn't see it. Mary, maybe he didn't say because he knew we would make him address it. He just succumbed to a disease far greater than any one moment. He was lonely. That was his cancer. Suicide is a great illusionist of rational thoughts."

"My family is devastated. All we can do is cling to each other. Why couldn't I help my brother?" she pleaded, sobbing.

"Mary, I offer this. In times when suicide becomes a devastating reality, perhaps who remains upholds life and each other with more care. You did everything right. We couldn't have seen this coming." I redeemed us all.

Mary gave her regards to her God almighty and thanked him for her strength. I thanked her for her valor and for the courtesy of the call and conversation.

We hung up and I sat resting the next patient clipboard on my chest. In that moment, I hated my job. I hated the burden of fighting battles I cannot fully see and being left in a war-torn, wounded family. I hated my failures to not see deep enough into a soul. I hated my cowardly downward gaze. I hated that we cannot see the real crisis that kills. I hated feeling alone against it all. I hate the responsibility of one problem that seemed to ignore the wholeness of a person. I hate my fallibility and the arrogance to stand up and enter another room despite it.

Then I got up and went into another room, starting all over.

♥

Add-on

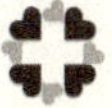

In the long stretch of a winter season that was swelling to a seismic storm, a request came to urgently add to my schedule a patient. Like a surprise pregnancy, the next day seemed to grow with reckless regard for me.

"Book him at 7 a.m. tomorrow," I sighed, exacerbated by the lack of Godlike powers to create time but burdened by a duty to serve a never-ending deluge of needs. The next day I would be asking my husband and children to understand why I had snuck away at 4 a.m. and did not say good morning before running to the hospital to round and then haphazardly racing to meet up with someone else's idea of "too early in the morning" at the office. Though I had learned years earlier that my son did best getting a long hug and a gentle reminder each morning to "focus" and "resist the urge to question every little thing for sake of time," my son would have to try reminding himself. I silently hoped his day would not be derailed by the seating arrangement contested or math class distracted by shenanigans untethered. The dread of a phone call from school fed an ever fear of being a poor mother and nurtured a corresponding resentment for duties as a doctor like water and sun sowing a seed in a styrofoam cup.

The night passed anxiously, as I organized time over and over in my head like a general readying for combat. The morning arrived and I left my home as the single soul awake venturing out into the darkness. Mercy was shown as I blew through the hospital, with every patient a sheer pleasure to meet. Problems were solved without a hitch, and the gates flung open to sail straight to the stranger added on. By 7 a.m. I was poised at my desk, already sorting insurance approvals and medication renewals.

The add-on checked in.

"His son is kind of angry," my medical assistant alerted me as she passed me a chart. The weight of the alert to be wary of balancing a second soul in the room exacted a brief shoulder sigh of acquiescence. I obeyed the design and straightened up to walk into the exam room. I promised silently to slow down and serve.

"They always are if they are feeling frustrated and impotent," I replied.

I entered the room and made fast work of the orientation. The add-on was ninety years old, and his oxygen concentrator clicked and bled out to a heart rate paced at sixty-five.

His son sat to the left, red-faced and arms folded. He had been just recently irritated and the skin lay prickled, disrupting the air around him. I shielded myself from the radiation of his abating fury and directed my attention to his father.

The patient's kidney function was slowly inching into a gray zone of discussions and decisions.

"Are you feeling well?" I asked.

"These last months I've been more tired," he admitted.

The dad had been eating less, lacking an appetite. His weight was fairly steady, and the stores of protein in his body slid slowly down. Nothing was too alarming, but here we were to regroup and determine our goals of care. His memory was waning. He was determined to live unbothered alone in an assisted facility, protesting every gesture of assistance.

"I get along fine," he maintained.

The son adjusted as if to interrupt and interject details of his efforts and explain their failings, but I spoke directly and rapidly and again shielded my agenda from augmentation.

"Dialysis is growing to be a consideration that we must explore," I explained.

We drove around all the hows and whys and whens. The dad absorbed what he could. I supplied recommendations based on his personal dilemmas and deliberations and also shared facts that told of the compromises a ninety-year-old would venture paying the hard tax of living dependent on dialysis. At ninety years of age, being on dialysis becomes almost always living with eighty percent tax and not enough "income" to live off of.

We parked at his assertion of DNR and DNI and idled around the question of whether to ever engage dialysis or not.

With some hard-won rapport, like terms of an arranged marriage, I squared away myself to my patient and apologized. "I have to ask you directly something." He nodded and readied, shifting his hips.

"So," I sought to seal, "would you choose to do dialysis to extend your life if your kidneys fail fully or you fail to thrive with what little function you progress to having over the next year?"

There was not even the essence of a noted pause in the room.

"No," he quickly answered, and his son adjusted in his seat, no longer upset but now reduced to a mere boy, someone's son. Even the son's mustache softened. He hated to hear the truth but did not disagree. His father voiced a finality, on the other side of which was no father to connect with.

"Okay. Just so you know I think you've made a very mature and intelligent decision. Also, it is not so unnatural. Culturally we think we must fight everything. If this was Europe, we would just gladly slow and ease ourselves into a walk and a tea and a siesta. America is not so gracious about death," I validated.

"So," the son stirred, already shrinking in his vinyl chair as if his feet dangled, "let me ask you. I call him every day and ask if he's eaten. I go every week and ask if he has taken his pills or filled his pillbox. We . . . we fight a lot and I . . . I just want to know what I'm supposed to do."

The sun was setting in the West over a world that was coming into focus, and a blade of grass was asking the sun what it should do through the night and till the morning.

"Let's ask your dad," I decided. "Sir, does it bother you to have your son nag you or help with pills?"

The son was not prepared for my antics or choice of words and tensed at the word "nag." On his lips were the readied protesting words, "See! See how he is difficult?"

"I'm fine with it," the dad assured.

I smiled a little at his simplicity.

"I guess it's not him but rather it's your frustration perhaps at an imperfect situation made hard by his choice for isolation and independence and frankly his poor memory. I think you reminding him is loving, is conversation, but be careful. Reminding someone who is forgetful can be frustrating and shaming and truly unproductive," I offered.

"I've started actually to back off," the son admitted with relief. "So, let me ask you something. We are leaving for the summer and . . . do you think that's a bad idea?"

I considered it and grimaced a bit to think everyone gone for months. "It would be fine except . . ." I started and the father finished by interjecting, "I'll be fine."

"I know," I agreed, "but, how about someone checking in, not to nag or touch anything but to wave at you twice a week?"

"I'll be fine," he repeated.

"Okay. But would you do it for your son to be fine and not worried?" I pleaded on his son's behalf. "Sometimes things are done for peace of another's mind. Plus, sir, if say something happened, your son would be left with guilt and self-loath that he had left you or let you talk him into leaving you alone."

The dad softened now. His oxygen seemed to sizz slower, and then he inhaled and nodded acceptance.

"So we actually tried it last week," the son offered. "The facility just had this free trial and we tried it."

"Oh! How was it?" I inquired.

"He didn't really like it," the son deflated.

"Sir, did it bother you," I asked.

"I'm fine," he replied and looked down to the left. The way he addressed me, I knew a secret.

"Sir," I rephrased, "do you recall anyone coming to check on you last week?"

"No," he clarified.

"There's your answer!" I concluded. "Arrange the service to merely check on him. He answers the door and visits a bit for good measure but doesn't truly recall the intrusion."

I then rolled over to the dad. "Sir, I want to tell you a story. Last week I was caring for a man. He is sicker than you. We were talking of many things and eventually he said he had a horrible holiday."

The dad nodded at this not-so-uncommon comment. He was surprised as well to consider someone sicker than himself.

"The thing was, he told me at some point he was with family and everyone was talking past him and despite him and without regard to him. Eventually hurt and frustrated he yelled, 'Hey! I'm right here!' Sir, I'm sorry if at any point you might have felt us talking about you and not to you. This was *your* appointment. This was our chance to understand you and best serve you."

The dad nodded approval and thanks and I rolled back.

The son shifted at this exchange and then it happened.

He added on.

"I have to apologize," he confessed. "Before when they brought us in they asked for my father's medicine list. I had typed it up and placed it in his wallet, but this time it was gone. I was so mad and irritated I asked my dad, 'Dad, where's the list I typed up? Why isn't it in there like it's supposed to be?' I said it very harshly and I used poor words. Dad . . . I'm sorry for that."

The room was center stage on ninety years of life totaling up.

The dad nodded in a proud and solemn way. His whole charge glowed a deep yellow. "This is *my* son."

"Come on, Dad. Let's go," the son gathered.

I hoped my son would have an uneventful if not special day. I had traded his needs for another son's needs.

My heart swelled as I watched them toddle down the hallway while I reached for the next door. My son would hear a story one day of why I had not said good morning one day in February when he was young. Maybe the many mornings we traded would come into focus, woven in his making and forgiven in time by the sonder attested in these stories.

♥

The Gray Zone

Outside the room where nurses were whispering loudly but respectfully, she waited. She was surrounded by taller and older aunts and uncles. The women clucked in their thoughts like hens, and the men said their peace boldly and then walked away like coyotes on a prowl, returning to the circle after a lap to distance themselves. She stood in the midst of all this chatter and swirl and felt dazed. The suddenness of all the most horrible realities was overwhelming.

I rushed back to the hospital, having gotten a call about a young lady sixty-three years old found down, arrested, then successfully revived after forty-five drawn-out minutes of touch and go. Shirley was now acidotic. I reviewed the most important facts and then called to speak to the daughter en route. I had to work quickly and needed to gauge the daughter and her ability to decide. I wanted to give her time to consider and digest what I didn't have to offer. While I drove in, we talked by phone.

"What was your name?"

"Katherine," she replied softly.

Katherine, daughter and medical power of attorney, steadied herself on the phone.

I inhaled to begin the litany of explanations that would grow increasingly esoteric.

I introduced myself and reviewed what I knew about how her mom had come to the hospital and was now currently intubated, on medicines to keep her blood pressure from plummeting and a special infusion of bicarbonate to help correct her blood pH.

"Katherine, there are ongoing issues evolving. She has organ failure, and from what we know likely brain damage. If you want me to try dialysis I can, but I am not sure she can handle it or if it will help. She is unstable and long-term has poor prognosis for recovery of any kind," I said against the noise of my turn signal and the cars around me. I drove the car habitually so all my attention was on speaking new facts.

"It . . . It happened so fast . . . She asked for a breathing treatment. My aunt . . . My aunt went to get it and then returned, and she was slumped over. But . . . she did this in April. She came in and spent one day in the ICU, then she did okay and went home . . . she went home then," Katherine stammered as she tried to sort events.

That event in April was similar indeed. Shirley was an admission for a COPD exacerbation, then an aspiration pneumonia that deteriorated to being intubated, but never did she arrest. This time she was at home when she played out the affair and capped off what was otherwise a repeat with an arrest. This time . . . she had brain edema. I sighed to highlight the difference as it would pain Katherine. Katherine heard me sigh. I felt badly. Katherine would not know the meanings of my sighs. She might feel suddenly judged or condescended. I wanted to explain to protect her. I sighed because I would have to tell Katherine boldly the difference between that prior time, home free, and this time, brain swelling and body failing. I pulled out the harsh-sounding and sternly striking reality stick my words can become and pulled back to swing it at Katherine. I did not want to beat her with my words. I put the proverbial stick down. I would not beat into Katherine the fact that her mother was dying.

"Katherine," I softened, driving past a turn and circling around again as if lost, "this is different."

I gave her an ETA and told her to think and talk to the family and I would be in to look at her mom. "I am coming," I assured, then hung up.

Focused on just driving, I fell into Katherine's shoes, then Shirley's, then the family I heard gathering in the background of our conversation. I felt my way around the way the narrative needed to go. The turn signal clicked, my empathy around the room laid out in my mind's eye in the dimensions that unfold within siblings, offspring, strangers, and medicine. *Turn left at the sister. Go. Turn right at the brothers. Go. Turn and park by the daughter. Rapidly gain trust like a long lost but easily relatable half-sister.*

I arrived at the throes of Shirley becoming hypotensive again. As the nurses and critical care doctor swiftly assessed and dosed more bicarbonate, I sought to find Katherine.

"Katherine?" I asked of one and then another woman I saw worrying at a drawn curtain.

"She's over here!" The nurse threw a wave to the left over to a gathering of family corralling uncertainty.

The circle opened and there Katherine stood. She had that childlike look in her eyes we all get when our moms are sick. She had been crying, and her hair was tied back in an exhausted fuss. Strands of hair flew all over. Her t-shirt didn't match her shorts. She had dressed in a panic. Her dry lips contrasted with her wet eyes. She had cried herself dehydrated in the wasteland of grief.

HEENT: head spinning, conjunctiva injected, ringing noises blaring out in a high-pitched tone, and the dehydrated skin choking her neck and forcing a lump in her throat

"I spoke to you on the phone. I'm Dr. Robey. I am the nephrologist on call," I introduced. I shot immediately into the now, having little time for her to choose me or not to choose me.

"Your mother is coding right now. Her pressures are dropping. We are trying to restabilize her. If we can, I need to know: Do you want me to try to dialyze her? It may not work. It may not even be possible if she gets again hypotensive. Do you want me to try?" I pressed.

A tall, barrel-chested man stepped forward and said, "If she can't wake up and walk home, let it go."

The group mumbled in agreement.

A very short white-haired woman with a cane and a head tremor stuttered. "If she's not going to wake up . . . Let it go."

I heard a nurse shout, "Okay, we have a pressure now!"

I turned and asked Katherine again, "Do you want me to try?"

Katherine glossed over. I imagined my voice sounded muffled to her, and the tone—like a high-pitched flat line—rang in her ears.

I touched her across what felt like an icy chasm.

My voice drowned back for her as she focused her eyes to a moment she was simultaneously running from.

> *"There is a feeling of disbelief that comes over you, that takes over, and you kind of go through the motions. You do what you're supposed to do, but in fact you're not there at all."*
>
> —Frederick Barthelme

"Katherine," I said, as I was talking over the business in the room. Her daze did not reach out for the rope thrown to her as she lay adrift. "I know because your mom did something like this before and because she is young and it all happened suddenly it feels gray but it is not gray. Her ability to survive meaningfully makes this black and white," I said. I wanted her to be okay with a decision to stop now and in the next week and in the next eternity after. Long after decisions are made, the memory of decisions gets twisted and haunts us with would-haves and should-haves.

Katherine put her hands on her head and pulled her hair and face tensely back. "Okay," she said.

I felt the ambiguity.

"Okay, what?" I thought but dared not say such an antagonizing thing. The unavoidable time had come and for sake of clarity I had to beat Katherine with the your-mother-is-dying stick.

"Katherine, your mother cannot survive this. She is dying. Do you want me to tell them to stop?" I asked.

But before she could answer, her mom was restabilized just on the brink of disaster and that left nothing to stop.

The gray zone set in.

The fact of the brain edema was minimized in light of this new brief stability gained with the eighth ampuls of bicarbonate.

It was too early in some mandatory heroism for the team to stop. It was too early for Katherine to see straight and command they stop. The family got swept away with trying again and brief interludes of mediocre calmness by comparison to a ravaging code. The idea of trying everything was logged, coded, and revived. The decision was made to dialyze Katherine's mother. The dialysis line went in and my dialysis nurse flew in as I typed and dictated. I finished my note, and another ampul of bicarbonate was called for. Shirley became stably unstable, but I could not confuse Katherine more to explain that inherently tenuous state.

Dialysis started forty minutes after I arrived in record time. Only in training where we all slept in a broom closet awaiting tragedy could we discuss, decide, thrust a line in, and dialyze this fast. I was happy it could play out fast. I felt reactive. I was certain I would fail but I had to fail while crawling out of the gray zone to the fresh stench of black. I wanted Katherine to feel reactive and fast even if she was growing to understand the futility of efforts.

My best dialysis nurse was on call and when he arrived he was lighthearted and agreeable. I was grateful for the cynicism because I could not handle the grief without this drug. I had texted him en route. "Oh, by the way, I know she has brain edema." Nephrologists are known to dialyze the near-dead. I did not want that reputation. Dylan knew I dialyze the living. Dylan knew I was dialyzing Katherine, her family, and our team. I had sent the text anyway because I felt wrong. I felt the gray zone choking me. I hoped he would not spread a rumor about me losing my clinical judgement.

He replied, "Miserably is the only way to fail."

Two hours into a slow high-bicarbonate run, Shirley became maxed out on four pressors with a blood pressures bowing down in the 70s.

> *"Death comes for us all; we can only choose how to face it when it comes."*
>
> —Robert Jordan

Given the gift of time to acclimated, Katherine asked to call it quits. At that permission, the team allowed the white elephant to be seen. Katherine had seen the commotion rising for the fifth time and said softly, "It's okay. You all can stop." As I was on the phone listening, I saw the layout with Katherine surrounded by her elders, still oddly feeling alone while bearing a decision to quit. I realized I should have just told her I would bear it and not dialyze her mom. I should have just said no to the moment myself. I realized I did her both choice and harm by not being more maternal in advice. The gray zone had infected my judgment after all.

Perhaps saying no to the moment for Katherine would have made us enemies. Perhaps Katherine would have written the narrative that I had refused her mom a chance to try. Perhaps that would have been short mercy for Katherine but long-term adversity with the world of medicine and doctors. Either way, the arms of the gray zone like death itself pulled at Katherine and drew her into the sticky pool of impotence and guilt. Either way we sank in the sludge of damnation doing or not doing together.

"God has mercifully ordered that the human brain works slowly; first the blow, hours afterwards the bruise."
—Walter de la Mare

"It all happened so fast," Katherine reeled in the quiet of heavy decisions made in the center of a circle of hens and coyotes.

The gray zone lay like a blanket over the mother in the bed. From that late afternoon over five hours, Shirley was dying and there was just not enough time to make it feel properly black and white.

I could not help but call Katherine to testify.

"Katherine," I said, as if her name called her back to reality with strength. "It was black and white. You did everything just perfectly. I am sorry. It happens this way sometimes. Let the gray darken."

Darkness fell as every monitor was turned off.

"While I thought I was learning to live I have been learning to die."
—Leonardo da Vinci

For days after, I wished I knew better how to instruct others to watch dying without misery and weariness. Sometimes there is no true contrast to call closure upon except that which doctoring can elucidate, taking the ownership of heroic efforts for the sake of dignity. Even then, doctoring falls victim to the fight that says we were once living and deserving of living.

♥

Sew Me a Story

My mother-in-law worried I would write a story about her full of sorrow and sadness. She worried as her mind slipped that she had told me something already and felt embarrassed, sensing something familiar but not completely.

Chances are . . .

Every day I wait for a chance. Chance arrived on a Tuesday as a lovely lady telling me stories in exchange for my medical analysis of her bloodwork. She had grandchildren that she giggled about. She was proud to have grandchildren.

"Here's the picture," she shared, presenting a perfectly preserved black and white image of a young lady and three children, all dressed alike in white pressed tops and plaid patterned suspendered dresses.

She had widowed with three young children, and in desperate times she had fought to clothe her children.

"These are the feed sack dresses I told you I sewed. Three cents a feed sack. Then the tops I made from flour sacks. Oh my, those outfits saved us but were such a pain to iron," she reminisced.

Chances are . . .

She remarried and that man adopted those three children. Together they moved to a home "with indoor plumbing," she regaled.

In the car to pass the time I chatted aimlessly to my mother-in-law about my day. I told her about the lady I had chanced that day who had widowed young, whose children preferred the outhouse with two holes rather than the toilet they eventually had indoors because they could not go if it were occupied and "had to wait."

"Oh, I know those days," my mother-in-law nodded.

"So she told me one visit about these feed sack dresses she made, Mom, and today she brought in a picture," I marveled.

Then my mother-in-law sparked a story I had never heard. "Oh, I had a feed sack dress," she shared.

Chances are . . .

I have not heard every story you could tell me, Mom, and I do not mind hearing all many, many times for as long as you are here to tell them, like a feed sack refurbished and a life that seems a waste of time anymore being a victim of dementia except you are full of surprises still.

♥

Responsorial

I. The Weight That Stays

"She should die sometime today," the astute and solemn decree fell. And yet, the long shadow of the sun fell instead across the room and rose again on the opposing wall day after day. She did not eat or stir or drink or speak. Yet, they said each day, "Today looks like the end."

"But she can hear us," the daughter-in-law surmised by some tremble of eyelids and some grasp of hands on theirs.

Days before, I received a notification that after ninety-three years, Mrs. Tanway had folded into hospice. Her son had called me to let me know. This unexpected courtesy showed me a kind of respect and affection, which I returned fully by calling him back. He was not one for words, and so he had married well a woman who easily spoke their thoughts and feelings.

"She seems . . . to be lingering here," the daughter-in-law said, concerned.

"I find those that linger long past the failing body are spiritually struggling," I explained. "They have some guilt or regret or fear or last business. It becomes exceptionally hard to tell what it is that holds them here if they have dementia. Disorientation makes the time of conflict hard to pinpoint. A person they may have unrest with may have passed long ago, or the unsorted issue may have long-expired importance.

There is some . . . secret or lasting wound troubling their soul. There is a weight that stays."

"I believe this!" the daughter-in-law exhaled. "Months ago, Danny asked his mom if she was afraid of dying and she said yes. He asked why and she said she didn't know where she would go after. She worried she would not go to Heaven. She was a very angry person for a long time and directed that anger often at many people. She can't even recall who or when or exactly what she did, but she feels badly now and gets everything mixed up."

The damning fear of karmic uncertainty felt frigid to Mrs. Tanway. Her thin nightgown would not bear the bone-biting wind of Hell surely coming. The looming uncertainty of what was next made staying lingering preferable. A cold eternity existing past the ninety-three years of earthly walking self-righteously and callously seemed a just oblivion, spent nameless, hopeless, and lonely. "I could go nowhere or go to Hell," Mrs. Tanway had told her son. Her scared and shamed soul hung ten stones around her bony neck and laid twelve stones upon her chest to counter the rise till she choked and wheezed but would not die and ascend anchored to Earth.

II. The Weight Lifted

"I find it intriguing that you feel she can hear you. I find this perfect, that perhaps you or her son or a chaplain can provide words of forgiveness or blessings. Can you rebaptize or rebirth her spirit? Would you find it helpful to provide her spirit with the release it needs? I ask because her soul has a weight and needs unbinding," I reflected.

"Yes, yes it would help, I think." Her daughter-in-law tingled.

"Perhaps, too, it would help you and your husband to try," I added.

"Yes, yes, it would feel good to us too," her daughter-in-law released.

They had the chaplain come and pray into Mrs. Tanway's ear and bathed her forehead in a cool, blessed bath, baptizing her anew. Then they waited more.

The sun rose, rolling back a stone that resurrected hope, and in three days' time she passed as the long shadow of the sun laid at last on her last sunset. Her eyelids ceased trembling. Her hand fell to the side, relaxed. The weight of staying became zeroed upon forgiveness, and she floated away. The body fell as minerals and mead to decay in a way that was not heartbreaking but affirming for those to come even if they came clumsy and at times cruelly. She was peaceful and that peace promised those coming that all was worth it and all was forgiven in the end if forgiveness was asked.

Often I am asked, "Doctor, how long? How long before they pass?"

We are but three things for certain: mortal, seeking peace, and answering our own profound inquiry, "What was the purpose of my life?" For these three shared truths, every story sounds like a story of dying but is rather a story of seeing one's living fulfilled and come to pass in forgiveness, not judgment.

♥

Readied

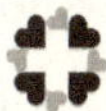

I did not have time to read the chart. I always go into a room knowing the playbook. I did not have time because I was leaving the hospital while already late for office. I turned around in the elevator and headed straight back to the room, where the new consult was waiting.

The husband sat at the foot of her bed. The daughter at her side. The patient lay under a heap of blankets. I had but the most rudimentary labs to explain my presence.

"Her labs indicated some potential issues with her kidneys," I said, defending my nosiness.

I asked how she felt. Her answers were slow and vague. She passed a majority of the review of systems but failed the ultimate sustainer. She was anorexic and at times had issues swallowing. She did not eat much. She did not drink much. She was swollen all over. She breathed short and shallow but slow and steady. Her husband launched into the greatest summation a lay family member ever delivered. "She had melanoma five years ago. She had the cancer completely resected and was cancer free until months ago they found some lymph nodes on a surveillance imaging. Those lymph nodes were biopsied and indicated return of melanoma. She had those radiated. Tomorrow they hope to remove the mass they finally found in her small intestine that has been causing blood loss," he summarized.

"What is the mass?" I asked, fully clueless.

"It is melanoma. In fact, the melanoma is everywhere now. It is in the lungs, liver, brain." He sorrowed and she sighed, and the daughter turned away.

I had seen this playbook.

They came to whisk the patient away for a transthoracic echocardiogram, and the husband asked to speak to me alone so I obliged him. It turned out, he merely wanted me to know her right leg always had swelling, for she had denied it when asked in her embolic delirium.

"Sir," I dared, "I have to ask you. It seems premature, but does she have a living will that tells us what to do if her heart stops or she stops breathing?"

He stood there sheepishly contemplating something, and I could not help but stare at his shirt pocket because out of it rose a pen and a plastic spoon and knife. I was mesmerized by the preparedness while he lamented about how they had just discussed these scenarios but had not yet signed the papers officially. "If she—we, for that matter—are terminal, we are DNR and DNI," he verified.

"Would you each elect for a feeding tube?" I pressed.

"No, ma'am," he answered frankly.

"You know, not in the imminent sense but in the broad truth your wife is terminal." I grabbed him firmly. "I know it sounds premature, but I have to be direct because if she is this swollen and this compromised and not eating and doesn't want a long-term feeding tube, then surgery tomorrow will result very quickly in moments that require you to draw very hard lines and/or stand by the ones you have drawn. She will have an impossible time coming off the ventilator post-op, and the volume she obtains peri-op will be such a horrible thing to get off with such poor nutrition. Post-resection she won't be able to eat, but she isn't eating now when most able by comparison. Without stable intake the issues become disastrously complex, and you suddenly find yourself executing those hardline decisions." I flashed forward. "I'm sorry to go so far ahead, but I want to be prepared with you and to protect you from those who also come questioning more urgently and therefore more harshly," I explained apologetically.

"I know," he teared up. "I don't think you're premature. I know. I . . ." he stumbled.

The spoon in his breast pocket slid next to the knife as he shifted and seemed to cling to the knife in a panic.

"I'm so sorry. You're just amazing to me," I worshipped, studying the moment, staring at his breast pocket. "Let's see what happens next." I bought him time to fully catch up to reality.

He nodded, heartbroken and slowly digesting what would soon be the weather forecasted.

"Sir, I have a question if I may, if you'll let me," I asked.

He nodded as he wiped his eyes.

"Sir, can I take a picture of your breast pocket with your spoon and knife sticking out?" I awkwardly asked.

He felt for his pocket, suddenly aware of cutlery in there, and laughed at himself. He agreed, amused. I quickly snapped the picture.

"Let me tell you why I'm so mesmerized by this. This whole time we stood here and talked, and you fought back tears and wanted to plan properly—the best hope for your wife with perfect things accounted for. I could not help but notice your pocket with the spoon and knife. I always carry a spoon in my purse in case I find food and haven't eaten, and I am losing steam. I plan for the invariable event that I'm trapped and hungry. You plan too. You come prepared. I know you plan. God love you for trying to plan for your wife. I love you so much for this."

He smiled and cried and then hugged me and our souls smashed. He started to sob, so I let him.

"I was a Boy Scout," he jested and let go.

"Never unprepared," I complimented. "It is hard to plan every scenario on paper. It is hard to take living wills and extract things like 'terminal' and 'never.' Likewise, it is hard to think too far ahead and not journey. It will be okay, but I apologize if I've gone too far past now. I just wanted to know if you're prepared."

He teared up more and then could not hold back the stream. He was finally at the true juncture, and from here he could see the peaks of futility. "I'm ready for that too now," he acquiesced.

I left him finally, hurrying to office to face the impatiently waiting. I left him to weather his day with his spoon and knife readied. I left him to contemplate where we were aiming so perhaps we would not go too far down the rabbit hole and find ourselves hungry for relief and tortured by empty efforts. I left him but would be back to journey more tomorrow with my spoon ready. I am not hopeless, but I am never unprepared for the harsh truth of our bodily limits and the limits of medicine to cure all things.

♥

Quilting

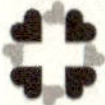

Cybil was not just anxious or afraid. She was suffocating.

Tracheal stenosis had gifted her with a tracheostomy. Diabetes had fated her on dialysis with a small portal for a window on this "pleasure cruise," as she was also vision impaired. She wore a new colorful scarf each time I saw her to cover the tracheostomy opening. She would place her finger over the opening of her tracheostomy to speak during exhalation, or was it a sighing I often could not distinguish? She was two hundred pounds overweight for her height, but she could walk still and that surprised many. Cybil always did her hair and smelled of sweet peas. From Maine to Arizona some ten years earlier, she and her husband retired. Her husband was a dentist now with mild dementia. She did all the talking. He did all the driving. She always came into the dialysis unit very flustered but never missed a treatment. She was having back pain because of sitting for so long, and in Maine she was placed on 4.5 hours as a standard run time.

I introduced myself one day as she was tethered to the dialysis machine.

"I was looking at your numbers and I actually think with your residual function I can drop you down to three hours," I said.

"Three hours?!" she exhaled, baffled and at last delighted. "That would be so much better!" as if finally a small reprieve was handed down to the life sentences she had served back to back. She gasped and exhaled out, "In Maine they never even negotiated. They just put me on and walked away. I'm a good Catholic girl, but sitting here after three hours makes me feel trapped." Her weight, her wheeze, her blindness, her kidney failure living on dialysis three times a week, her back pain made her feel hostage to her life.

Her shoulders relaxed over the next months, and she began to tell me a little about her life since I had gifted her a personhood. By the fourth month I had learned she never could have children but loved them deeply. She adopted three children. One was very feisty and would give the nuns at school a lot of "sass" but grew to be a very strong leader. Sarah was Korean but homegrown on French fries and milkshakes. "She is all American," she would beam. Sarah was their first but then came Mary and David. Sarah kept them in line.

It turned out Cybil had been a queen quilter before losing her sight. It turned out that her quilts were much sought after by all of Maine. When she arrived in Arizona she quilted Arizona sunsets. Not knowing much about quilting except squares interlinked, I tried to envision a sunset in squares. The way she spoke of quilting, I believed the square sunsets were beautiful and forgot the geometric impossibility.

One summer she was heading back to Maine. I thought she would be overjoyed. She was back to anxious and suffocated.

"Cybil, why are you stressed? I think you are okay to travel and all your labs look great," I asked.

"Dr. Robey . . ." She tensed up and looked like a school girl admitting something grave. "I called the unit I went to before, which Dennis knows how to get to, and they said they would run me there but would increase my time to four hours, thirty minutes again. I just can't do it. I'll fail."

"Why do they want to do that? You have been feeling great and your labs are spot on," I asked, bewildered and a little defensive.

"They say they run everyone all the same," she sobbed.

"But you aren't all the same and you shouldn't be discredited for having some residual function," I said, wondering if I had missed a national movement or critical study. It didn't matter. For Cybil, the last year had been renewed living and I was not going to lose that ground. "Listen. I looked at your labs. I think you are okay to run three hours. You'll be gone for a month only. How do you feel about being 'naughty' and running just three hours regardless of what they order?" I asked.

"I don't know. I feel . . . Wrong. I feel nervous that I would be labeled 'the bad girl.' They would tell me I'm going to kill myself or that I'll die. I can't bear that and then Dennis will worry," she fretted, exhaling rapidly to talk.

I grabbed her hand. "It will be okay. How about this? How about you try your best and do what you can as much as you can and don't worry so much?" I offered. "I think you will be okay either way."

She dried her tears.

That summer she was gone for a month. When she returned I found her elated and healthy.

"How was your trip?" I asked. She smiled, inhaled, then placed her finger on the tracheostomy hole and exhaled. "Amazing! I went into the unit like usual and at first I fell into the same fat, blind dialysis patient, but then I thought of what you said and I don't know—I just told them I was going to run for three hours only and they made me sign a form at first but then agreed to change my time after looking at my labs. They said since I was just visiting they would allow me to stay as I was here!" she sang.

"I'm so happy for you! I'm glad you spoke up. I'm glad you are doing well and feel in control," I said, sharing her renewed sense of self and control.

We were both smiling all day.

She did this for two summers and was with me the rest of each year. She seemed to own her life again. Dennis was getting more demented and soon could no longer could drive. There was worry he might be having seizures.

"Dennis is just not clear in the mind anymore," Cybil exhaled and sighed, sighed and exhaled.

Time marches strangely when you watch the ill or old. It becomes obvious that time starts rolling down a hill at some point.

One day Cybil developed a cough and fever. Within a day she was in the hospital, septic with pneumonia. She required two pressors and was on the ventilator for the first time in twelve years.

I came into her hospital room, and she awoke to find me holding her hand. She couldn't speak anymore, but her eyes welled up and the ventilator alarmed as she tried.

"Hi," I said, looking at the quilting queen. "You feel okay?"

She nodded yes and then looked down and to the left.

"You feel trapped again?" I assessed.

Her eyes grew wide and she nodded vigorously. She squeezed my hand.

"I heard your children are coming," I said.

She smiled and looked up into the heavens with eager anticipation. We played charades for another fifteen minutes and then I left.

The next day her room was filled with people. She was sleeping but her husband was at the bedside and three other adults were standing in the room: Sarah, Mary, and David. There they were. Sarah was a short Asian lady with a sharp bob. Mary was a brunette, lean with glasses. David was a blond with fairer skin whose cheeks seemed forever flushed. There they were. They were a surprising assortment of children, so much like a sunset. Strikingly different yet tied to this lady in bed by bonds of motherhood. I felt overwhelmed by beauty. By the idea that love could gather anyone and bind them. I saw these two people married but childless and diligently gathering a family from dark corners that had been filled with notions of unwantedness. I saw a family and loved how my stupid prejudice questioned who all the adults were, but the narrative I knew attested exactly their beloved status.

"Dr. Robey," Mary started, "we have heard so much about you."

"Dr. Robey." Sarah shook my hand gratefully. "My sister and brother are so happy to meet you finally."

"Dr. Robey." David took my hand like a lifeline.

The phrase "my sister and brother" lingered in the room and in my mind till I felt I would explode with joy. *Oh, my quilter queen! Look at what you made,* I thought. *You quilted a family.*

Cybil was waking. I walked to her bedside, nodded, and said hello to Dennis and then greeted Cybil.

"I just met your kids," I said.

Cybil looked around the room, likely only seeing blurs, then smiled.

"They are all like you said they would be," I smiled. Like characters coming alive from a storybook, her children presented themselves and I was flooded with wonderment.

Sarah spoke now. "Dr. Robey, Mom feels tired. She's been thinking . . . about stopping dialysis." Behind her, her sibling created a second to the call to a vote.

I had to apologize for my smile. "Sarah, your mom said you were the take-charge one. Direct with nuns. Fearless with truth," I said. Cybil's laughter set the ventilator alarm off.

The children eased and laughed.

I addressed the room. I addressed Cybil. I addressed the children. The children were adults and reasonable and loving. No major hysterics or drama. They all seemed calm, considerate, and grateful. "I'm so glad I met you all together. Your mother is so proud of each of you," I said. The children left with their dad, then I spoke with just Cybil.

"Cybil, they are just as you said they are," I beamed. We were two girls gossiping. Cybil mouthed, "I know!" and we laughed together. The ventilator shushed us.

A pause as the ventilator quieted.

"Cybil, are you really ready to rest?" I asked, serious now.

Cybil nodded.

"Cybil, I'm so proud of you. I think you have come a long way into a happier life since I met you. I have enjoyed your stories, and now having met your children I have felt this awesome joy. It's like a book coming alive. How you must think it is funny for me to meet them and be so in awe," I said, starting to tear up.

Cybil started to cry, but she looked resolved and at peace.

The final threads were placed on a perfect quilt, and a beautiful sunset appeared in what were squares to us.

Cybil passed that night.

Weeks later, alone, her husband made his way to my office. He presented me with a beautiful hanging quilt of purple, orange, yellow, and red waves quilted in very asymmetrical designs. A black cactus was amid swirls of patchwork colors. Signed on the bottom was "Cybil Bergeron." Here was the winning quilt of 2006. One of the last Cybil made before she lost her eyesight.

Amazing what is in our souls. How these things find their way to the world. Cybil the quilting queen quilted for three a life where only uncertainly had lain. Made them all a family. Knew their souls. Sewed together illnesses, care for a spouse, travel, and self-growth, and made a little patch for me and my journey.

Then . . . she passed on.

I imagine she is someplace speaking without being breathless and never anxious and smelling of sweat peas. I wonder what she will do with all those colorful scarves. Then I see the sunset and know she's quilting them into the sky for all to see.

♥

A Yellow Wood

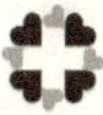

"Two roads diverged in a wood, and I—I took the one less traveled by, and that has made all the difference."

—Robert Frost

Over the last four years, his anxiety increased and he became easily frustrated.

"Now if you would just listen to me," he would insist. I had my days when I would retort, "I am listening to *you* and I'm hearing you."

At ninety-plus, he was frustrated by what he saw as failures of mine or the system, but it was actually just his world closing in with limited easy solutions.

Today he was my second to last patient. He did not tax me one bit, even though limited time threatened to set me on edge.

I flung the exam door open without knocking, as was my manner. The office had become my other home and these exam rooms like bedrooms and sitting rooms in an efficient residence. There they sat in the ten-by-six-feet space that opened up like an expanded hall: Mr. Frost and his bride of seventy years along with his daughter, a nurse, and her husband as supporting cast. They all startled a bit except for him, for he could not hear a dump truck interrupt. I broke the power imbalance created by my entry without knocking by immediately acknowledging the wife, whom he honored but I had never met.

"I've heard a lot about you," I beamed.

The way he had spoken of his need to live long to care for his wife, I thought her to be frail and needy. She sat composed, and as she spoke to tell his woes and her concerns, I was enamored and enthralled.

"Tell her, Mom, what you have seen," the daughter invited.

I set to typing like a legal recorder, and Mrs. Frost allowed it as I complimented the tempo of her tales with rhythmic clicking. The sound of music piped into my mind like a movie set to a soundtrack.

She started, and midway through the telling of the evolution of her beloved husband's undoings of late, he interrupted. "Now, Doc," he commanded, "I need you to listen to my wife because I'm going to let her tell you what she sees from her eyes."

I just nodded obedience while typing away, but over my left shoulder I felt his daughter recoil that I might be offended by the bizarre need to interrupt what was already engaged. Then the tension behind me relaxed as I allowed myself to be perceived as even needy and eager for commanding.

The wife escalated the ways Frost had unraveled of late, and in the end I nodded more vigorously. He was layering uremia on his dementia, and kidney failure's consequences were upon him. Her natural pause invited my jump into the explanation and possible solutions.

Seeing that he could not hear or follow well, I asked them to scoot in closer and watch me draw the possibilities onto the exam table cover torn off to use as paper.

As I spoke, I drew a line and a little sedan atop the line. Next to it I wrote, "Home. Comfort." Then I drew a line jutting the opposing way, creating an obtuse angle. Atop that line another sedan driving away and the words "Three-times-a-week dialysis. Some better mental clarity. Chore. Fatigue."

Each line was the same length even without a ruler. Some part of my secondary brain disappeared to think on how many lines one must draw to become naturally equal ones without care.

I pointed to the juncture of the two lines meeting and announced, "You are here," like a mall map. Then I traced both journeys and asked which he wanted to travel.

The wife begin to speak and said for clarity, "If it was me," but I stopped her, gently touching the perfectly placed hand she had on the light and awkwardly torn exam cover we used as a roadmap, and added, "Can I tell you what he told me years ago was his motivation?"

She replied, "Can I tell you he said, 'To be around to care for my wife'?"

I smacked the table at our mutual understanding, then let her proceed given her veto power.

It quickly turned out at the yellow woods the wife wanted to be home, as they had lived an excellent life and it would do her best if he did not engage the hardship of dialysis to only fail and have her fail with him to bear that journey and to have him watch himself fail and see her fail him in some circle of pathetic elderly shortcomings. On dialysis, they would be tripping over rolled-up rugs left lying around a cluttered hallway just before life's back door.

"We have done it all. We have beautiful grandchildren. We have had everything." She teared up.

I looked around the museum of their life together and it was a gallery of joy.

I smacked the table again, speechless I admitted, because, "I owe my wisdom from decades of doing one thing well, and here you are, my dear lady, understanding naturally the juxtaposition and the truth of the choices we think we are making and the consequences we think we are enacting."

She turned to her husband, pointing to the little drawn sedan on the line with home and comfort in mind, and he nodded strong agreeance just as the day when they had signed to buy their first home together.

There was a little time for him given the details of his mind under uremic pressures, but not much. I folded up the drawing we had made together and offered it to the wife as reference and point of conversation later. She accepted it like a handkerchief, so light in her gentle clasps, and it lay irregularly folded.

"Do you want me to sign our Picasso?" I teased.

She opened her hands to give it to me again to do so, but I laughed and told her no—a hug was all I needed to sign off with.

I hugged her, hoping the smell of her well-perceived thoughts and satisfied living would coat me like so many powerful perfumes. She fell into my embrace with gratitude for my honoring her fully and for loving his funny ways.

To them all, I instructed, "Call me. Tell me how you've arrived at a decision. Call me and I'll help you situate," and we parted.

The door to the exam room opened and out flooded relief, mutual understanding, wild and hefty love, confidence, courage, support, choice, beauty, and this bride, whom I understood could move Heaven and Earth with her composure, strength, gratitude, and ease. She was not in need of anything but validation to not need anything. One would have heard the church organ play and a couple emerge married.

I turned to reorient my next mission when the daughter caught me and hugged me, and I fell into that hug, letting it hold us for a full thirty seconds.

"Thank you," she cried softly.

Two roads diverged in a yellow wood,
And sorry I could not travel both
And be one traveler, long I stood
And looked down one as far as I could
To where it bent in the undergrowth;

—Robert Frost

♥

Stretch

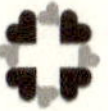

He was an understated man, but loyal. He came in once after a hospitalization that included urinary retention and renal failure. He checked in and I told him clearly he had significant impairment in kidney function after years of slow and undiagnosed prostate enlargement and urinary obstruction. He took in the details but left that day with other priorities. Dust seemed to settle around him differently; he was not interested in the very reality that was the hallway, the door, my verdict, his fate.

Under the advice of his urologist, he arrived again at my office. He had been gone for two years, and in that time prostate cancer had spread, defying the treatments. His kidney function had progressed, and now the oncologist asked the urologist to do more, and in turn I was asked to do more to reverse the failure and secure far more kidney function to engage a radioactive infusion. "He will need 30 percent function to best excrete the radiative substance. It is his only treatment option left," they said as they commissioned me, his nephrologist. Together we were the disciples of fate, and as fate would have it, Mr. Henderson was out of current options.

"How does my ultrasound look?" he perked up, eager to hear the verdict. He had devised a plan whereby I would "rig the kidneys and therefore open the pathway" to treatment.

"Well, fine except that is bad because we needed a fixable problem." I wrung my face out and looked down at the nothing left beside me, then to Mr. Henderson. "Mr. Henderson, I know you have these grandchildren at home. You told me about them the first time we met. How are they? How old are they?" I inquired.

I had stated their birthdays in my note. The countdown to when both grandchildren became eighteen years old relative to the clock to count the months left to survive metastatic cancer and bridge their adolescence was the movie composition to which the narrative danced to. Mr. Henderson had adopted them eleven years earlier when their mother became addicted to opioids. He promised them stability and delivered by picking them up from school and providing a home and meals. He divorced his second wife, choosing them over her, and he never regretted that choice.

"The eighteen-year-old has left but I still have the sixteen-year-old at home. I need . . ." He calculated and I interrupted to say, "One year and nine months by his birthday."

He paused at the awareness that I knew and had been actively calculating.

"Mr. Henderson," I drew out his attention, "we don't have that time. You are rapidly declining, and we are going to likely only have six months. I cannot get more out of your kidneys, and without them much better, you are not a candidate for the radioactive treatment. You need to hope for therapies to meet you in the future to survive to engage. Otherwise, we need to also call on more support and hope that more support also helps us extend your time. Who will care for your grandson if you pass?"

Mr. Henderson sat forward and offered his ex-wife and the children's mother. For now he maintained he would see to the grandson, as he had promised to eleven years earlier. He admitted it was hard to get out of bed or to eat, but he said he was determined to exact the "one year and nine months" he needed. "I am going to raise these kids," he repeated. "I am going to stretch this shit out," he swore.

We ended our visit with few options but a promise to me he would come back monthly to see anything coming that would itself be fixable. As he walked down the hall slowly, I saw the dust moving around him in a cautious fall that seemed to understand that his decisions operated on other laws. Some of the dust chose to evade him, and some dared to fall on him.

I thought to myself, *Could a man attempting to finish a good intention do it uninterrupted by mortality?* With that he opened the door and walked out, daring principles of fairness and justice to splint the breaks in his bones riddled with cancer.

♥

At First . . .

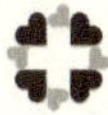

At first, she said she would not do it. She would not get the blood draws or temporary dialysis catheter or do dialysis.

At first, she said flat out, "No."

"But why not?" I pressed.

"Because I like to gamble, and this three-times-a-week thingy will ruin my Wednesday or Tuesday nights," she declared.

I felt tired by these words, like they vacuumed the air out of my lungs, but I pushed past the flimsy veil of resistance. "You're gambling now with your life, so please let us be realistic," I insisted.

"Fine," she acquiesced, and in three days she was humming along.

Discharged home, she entered the outpatient arena and began the ascension toward acquiring a better dialysis access and eating right.

At first, she did not like needles.

"I'm never getting that whatever you call it, fistula, because I can't stand needles," she scoffed.

"Well, I'll ask you every time I see you and offer you any number of tools to numb your skin as a trial," I compromised. "I'm just happy you're here with us and gambled correctly."

She made it to the casinos on off-dialysis days, and her granddaughter doted on her. She dyed her hair hot pink. She learned to laugh and goat us when she could about anything exposed worth taunting. We enjoyed her jabs as evidence she had the upper hand. She won thousands of dollars once at slots. We never heard about the losses.

At first, she missed an appointment to get the fistula created, but then she rescheduled and the surgeon took a picture of his handiwork to prove to me she went. He teased her about her pink hair and told her he liked her spirit. I thanked him for the added measure of cheering her on.

"I called her a pink she-devil," he shared.

"I bet she loved that," I thanked.

At first, she would not try any of our anesthetic, and then one day she barked an order at me, "Give me that spray thingy you always talk about. I'll try it."

"Yes, ma'am!" I jumped.

At first, she was impatient waiting to use the fistula and to get the catheter out. She sprayed her arm and pinched around to assure herself that when it was time she would be in control.

At first, we used small needles and she rolled her eyes at the lack of pain. Soon we were rolling down I-95 without a problem.

We advanced the needle size and churned away, and the catheter flew out along the side of our highway. Failure was a blur at 65 mph with pink hair blowing in the wind.

We were Thelma and Louise and we were roaring, leaving the loser boys behind and not letting anyone or anything beat us senseless again.

Then one month the ride was coming to an end. Just as quick as we were cruising, she fell and broke her hip and kept falling metaphorically. She could not swallow well and started eating less. The achalastic esophagus was killing her softly. Partly delirious, she refused any procedures and quite quickly she came to the end of the freeway under our construction. Her beautiful convertible flew off the cliff and her head scarf trailed behind her caught in the wind. I had rolled out of her car just before she grabbed air and watched her fly then fall out of sight as her pink hair smacked the blue sky. I waved to her and she seemed to still be fiercely screaming, "I just won't."

Goodbye, fierce Jacqueline. You made me at first so tired and then made me believe in vigor and the power of vinegar. May the slot machines in heaven all pay out.

♥

JJ

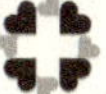

He had moved from another state. After eighteen years he came to me to roost. I thought him a funny guy. He always looked at me sideways until one day he said "Well, all right" to something I asked him to do. From then on he always replied the same pleasant agreeance.

He went in and out of an inpatient psych ward because of a mounting depression over being homeless, hopeless, lost, and lonely. One day I saw him in a room by himself looking out a window. His eyes were soft and thoughtful. "I don't know, Dr. Robey," he said. I touched his arm and told him swiftly, "You've been around this longer than I've been a nephrologist. Keep going, JJ." Each admission got longer because he had fewer and fewer options to discharge to. He was a little unwanted, but at my unit we idolized his resilience.

"Well, all right," he laughed at the comment that we admired him.

He finally landed at a place called Circle City. I feared he would just go around in a circle there. It was twenty miles away, and he waited often hours after dialysis to go home, but still he came to *my* unit.

He roosted. He would laugh at all our jokes. We fed him. One nurse made double portions for lunch and shoved half onto his plate as he waited for a ride that threatened to not pick him up.

By the end of 2019 we voted him "Student of the Year." His labs were not perfect, but he was a man who used what he had and never complained too much. He just was happy to belong somewhere. I left the unit midday in December and bought a large plastic trundle, three t-shirts, six pairs of socks, two button-downs, two polos, four boxers, and a lightweight jacket. I put it all in the trundle and left it for him. We at the dialysis unit try to help the helpless, and it was my thought suddenly that my days of helping JJ were ending. The thought fell into my mind with the click of the trundle closing and I felt the weight of last things done to give dignity before death comes to settle a life.

The day he was given the anonymous gift, the story goes, he fell to his knees, crying, "Thank you, Jesus."

Two months later COVID began to sweep the globe.

During the Covid crisis, JJ decided he would stop his circle and withdraw from dialysis, as he was now isolated from even the meager things he could connect to. I was beyond sad to know his time was ending. But it was his choice, and at least no one questioned his sanity. Twenty years on dialysis. I cannot name many things I have done for twenty years, but I have been married to one man for twenty years and I graduated medical school in 2000. My daughter turns twenty this year. Time is a moving element till it is not for us. Over the twenty years I cared for JJ it has been my honor to close out his every need I could.

"Well, all right," he would say.

When he died there was no one who knew him for me to call. I just wanted to tell you he existed. You should know he existed. If *he* could exist, we have no excuses. If someone acknowledged he existed, we might take care to always cherish existence lest we discredit our own relevance.

"Thank you, Jesus," he had exclaimed over a tub of nothing, and yet we fret daily with complaint in our throats in lieu of gratitude.

♥

The One Who Flew over the Cuckoo's Nest

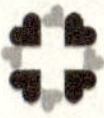

She was someone who would best me. I hated to accept it, but upon entering her world of tragedy and circumstance, I faced literally the ONE who would take me down.

"You know, caring for me will be trouble," she had warned years ago.

She would drop in randomly, demanding to be seen, and try to woo me with her words, impress me with her sly achievements. She knew, though, that I knew her secrets and kept them. She knew I kept away bigger wolves that dared drag her to justice. She knew I never lied, not to her or the wolves. The truth I spoke, the hope I swung, and the evil I shielded her from were tiresome and constant. My door was always calmly open. She evaded the law, yet evil took bites of her flesh. She called herself religious, but only the Devil seemed to answer her prayers.

"He raped you?" I worried. "They steal narcotics from you?" I furrowed. "You are sleeping on top of your purse?" I examined her when she complained of strange back pain. "Your parents want you to go back to your rapist so he can drive you to appointments," I flabbergasted.

The hostility of her birthright bore down on her. Her coping skills doubled down on generations of strife. She was easy to hate. Ironically, if it was not for her developed and defensive character of manipulation, I do not think I could care about her. I only cared about her to not succumb to the trigger she elicited to hate that would make me wrong and her a victim. I cared to not be accused of not caring and leave her leveraged over me. That is how good a con she was. She twisted things to survive, and her daughter was a cookie-cutter copy of her to likely breed the same.

"I don't know if this will work, but I will try," I asserted over and over when her circumstances pushed my creative problem solving skills. "You have to get on top of this. You have to make illness your bitch or it's going to do that to you," I charged once when she seemed genuinely a victim.

"Oh, I can be a bitch," she related. This I loved about her.

Rodeo after rodeo later, I knew what she was made of and she knew what I was made of. Frankly, we weren't so different.

"Dr. Robey, you have to try," she pleaded, twisting my words in a late phone call after hours till she made everyone "check with Dr. Robey," using my name in vain to create leverage and dissension. "You told me to make this *my* bitch. I'm trying. Please help me," she evoked. She had needs; she was growing blind with PRESS Syndrome. She had failings with friends who stole from her all around. I pictured her huddled atop her purse, batting at the air. "Who's there? Who is here in the room?"

Over and over I begged other physicians to help me do seemingly bizarre and dangerous things.

"I have never dialyzed a patient with a heart rate of 220," said the concerned intensivist once exclaimed.

"We will today. I have no choice," I held.

Over and over oddities to science and social services showed up.

"I have never seen such a dialysis access," I marveled. "Where did you find this home service?" I was astounded. "How often do they visit your home?" I admired.

There were parents, families, community, religion, and a child involved. There was a dangerous intertwined dependency with generational deceit validated on the need to survive. Damage was bled into the carpets and wallpaper. Every member of the household awoke unsure and distrusting but "God-fearing." They aimed to intimidate me, and only my confidence in my earnest efforts, good intentions, and obviously stretched patience and faith kept them from overpowering me with their blame. They hated me and said so outwardly.

"Dr. Robey, they want me to fire you," she challenged.

"What do you want?" I asked.

"I told them no. There is no one else," she maintained.

There was no one else. I was her third nephrologist. Leaving me, she would find herself stranded and finally alone and seen for the layers of black widowed weaves woven.

I warned everyone who met her to be mindful of their emotions for she could trigger a cascade of mistakes and poor acts. Then, I reasoned, they would swiftly be caught in half-truths and some fault.

The time came like an avalanche hitting the right frequency. She was given every inch at my bequest and advocacy, and she said, "No more. I'm tired."

Then she got even more allowances with magically arranged high-flow oxygen and pressors, and even more with chaplains escorting her home, and then somehow got home to die. I have never seen the things I saw caring for her. I have never seen medicine stretched into bizarre, creative, and unreal terrains. It was as if God came to save a wretch and chose her over every good soul to show he would save her too from being judged unworthy.

She taught me a kind of awesome admiration for the pure power in perpetuated evil. The profound awe at still the grace of God yielding to personhood, yielding to a human even if love hides in wicked caught only mid-blink. I hated her, but I did love how she made illness her bitch.

♥

Bones

The large pink sweatsuit swallowed her gray hair and pale skin. She seemed poised while walking steadily. I wondered why she would hide under such clothes. Perhaps it had been a lazy morning or busy time and she just threw on the heap and came in.

I sat nonchalantly, flipping pages and typing bits of my note, as her son sat hidden by the computer screen, asking me about his mother's laboratory results. It was the second visit, and we were wrapping up the workup. It all seemed quite benign. I saw her in the loud pink sweatsuit looking eager and interested. She looked like a huge bubble blown with bubblegum. I saw her in the corner of my left eye but heard him.

"Well, it all looks fairly okay. Your kidney function is mildly impaired. The cause seems mostly age and high blood pressure, which is controlled now. In my world, we must consider your age to calculate your ability to maintain what kidney function you have left to make it the rest of your journey. You are—" I stopped to glance at her chart. "—eighty, so . . ." I paused and turned to look at her directly. "You will be fine." I smiled. She would have an easy "60,000 miles" to head out into her nineties.

She seemed unimpressed.

"Okay," she replied. The pink sweatsuit was more excited by my news than she was.

I waited and returned to flipping more papers, scribbling and signing.

"I have this," she started, "thing, though. I'm on these medicines for depression, and the new one works pretty well, I think, but I have this thing where I suddenly wake in a panic. I'm not sure why but I just . . ." She stopped. I did not look at her as it seemed for a moment she needed to be seen but not looked at. "I just wake up gasping and panic."

I was flipping facts around in my head and papers in my hands with details of her and adding swiftly. Nothing about her screamed orthopnea or paroxysmal dyspnea, and so out of my mouth came, "I find that people who have such sudden grips of panic have had extreme trauma." I was not exactly sure where such a bold statement came from, but next she met me on the chessboard and moved her pieces even to mine.

"Yes. Well, my daughter was murdered forty years ago and I . . ." She started to suddenly cry. "I just don't want to talk about it."

Checkmate.

The son stared out the window now. I was grateful he had the window to leave from.

"Well—" I still did not look at her directly. "—you're talking about it now."

She told me more about the days and years after the murder.

"I didn't really grieve after because I was going to find the murderer. You couldn't stop me. If I was getting on a plane, then I was getting on a plane. Two years I worked but I found him." She was now a force, and her voice was strong and direct. I was amazed by the hot pink sweatsuit contrast because she pounded her words with such bold clarity. She was soft cotton candy with fists made of dense sugar.

I listened and then urged her to seek deep counseling. She refused and said she never wanted to talk about it. She was not going there. She cried softly, and the son stared more intently out the window.

"I think I inherited this anxiety and depression from her," her son said.

Time stopped. I put the papers away and then looked directly at her.

"Listen. Your kidneys are nothing to worry me. Your blood pressure, nothing to me. But I will tell you that what you cannot talk about, which you are talking about now with me, will come for you. If you live ten more years and then go to die, you will have a hard time leaving without a sense of peace. Also, what time you have left you will have little joy. You *need* to deal with this so you can have a few good years before you move on. Regardless, it will come for you. Trauma cannot be displaced and hidden. It does not wait quietly. It erodes the soul and stomps and is loud enough to wake you each night. You can use medicines to temper and balance, but you need to wrestle it directly in counseling. It will come for you anyway," I promised her. "It will murder you over and over again," I chilled.

She startled a bit at the direct and haunting words. I let her sweatsuit take shape around the reality, and her posture seemed better convicted against the undecided and amorphous heap of bright indifference. She did not say anything about agreeing to go to counseling. She said she had tried counseling before but found the process and people terrible and all a fit too hard to exact.

"I want a few good years," she mused.

"It will be extremely hard to talk about grief like this, but every day you don't address this, you choose living in her murdered days over living at all, and time is short. It will come for you anyway." I rose and hugged her. She hugged me back, and the bones of her body were hard and meatless. The sweatsuit hid her pains and bones, but somehow she had let me in and I promised her the fat and form would return to her if she merely addressed it. I promised her some cushion to ready her departure when she passed if she would just deal with the murder of her daughter.

"I'll still be here over the next twenty years and will see your passing. If you deal with this, I promise it will be a better time until and at the moment you must leave," I started to close.

She nodded but made no promises.

I started to clear and clean. "I don't think you will leave here and suddenly do anything but let it digest and know always that it will come for you. Head it off. Take it back. Get relief and control over the trauma. You hunted a murderer. Now it is time to hunt the pain down and dismiss it." We rose to part.

Death comes for us all. Those who live well and thus die ready deal bravely with the traumas of life as they come. It is paramount that we find and treat all diseases that lay in the way of living and passing, even the ones we do not see at first or are not particularly charged with addressing. Doctoring is daring to touch the bones of a problem despite the facade and texture we were initially presented with. If one doctors for a patient's lifetime, it behooves us to seek the source of dying while alive.

♥

Two Hours, Nine Minutes

Scientists argue over the merit of time. Most scientists understand time as a social construct and relative to forces like gravity and presence. If a person, being just matter, is not present then perhaps, some radically argue, no time passes or a lot of time passes, signifying the significance or insignificance of a person. Scientists, not social scientists or philosophers, question time. It is hard to imagine that a metric that is thought to be objective could carry little more than the pressure to measure once observed, lest we lose accurate track of it.

Telemedicine existed for decades born of rural care and a substitute for home visits, which became a rare feature of American medicine. It saves time. Sometimes it matters to matters like people.

He breathed into the receiver slowly and steadily. I regarded his speech as easy and free of halt. His wife laughed a hello to me and thanked me for a few callbacks and the urgent work via telemedicine. He had gained eight pounds in eight days and worried about his heavy legs. He was fifteen days shy of Christmas and had already taken a handful of medicines. He asked me for "possibilities" on a Friday afternoon.

"It depends what you're after. Likely, you have to come into the hospital," I argued. I ran the options, and all were already exhausted enough. Much more waiting at home with meager means would simply leave him on a Monday up two more pounds and none the wiser.

He sighed but did the math alongside me and hoped with fifteen days to play around with he could be better and home by Christmas. The wait in the ER was his biggest chore and waste of time.

He went into the hospital quicker than most for reasons not necessarily great to have. His cardiac enzymes pushed the midrange of triple digits, though never did he have pain. He sat as promised in a room with sterile decor and waited as medicine dripped in and urine spilled out. His biochemistry maintained on the edge of mischief, and questions arose as to the last of his heart's integrity.

"You appear to have had a major heart attack, and to know more or do more likely will place you on dialysis. As it is, you flirt with dialysis and to venture may only expedite a very drawn-out, dismal affair, weaker each day spent here. Should we gamble it all in the American way, or call it a draw and head home to siesta?" I asked on the third day of fifteen to kill.

I had only met up with him and his wife a total of two hours and nine minutes over the course of two months. So short a time to offer an opinion or company on a journey with decisions to be made. We stood on a precipice and looked over a deep and wide canyon, and we asked ourselves if *down* with an exceedingly slim chance of *out* was best. Or should we turn and walk on our own accord back to a place we had grown to see the story of on the back end of a life? He came into the hospital on a Friday afternoon with hopes of being fixed up, but instead was quickly positioned to face knowing why he was dying and to control how he might face it.

"I've lived a great life," he emphasized, not bitter or betrayed. He smiled and welcomed an end without tantrum or disgust. He looked over at his wife, who was neither dramatic or pale, and she said frankly as well, "We talked about this, and we know what we would do if this time came."

They nodded in unison, and the clock clicked off a second in an illusion of time to their head folding forward and another click for their heads rising back up. Then time stopped, and a gaping hole opened into a black vortex as he looked at me.

"I never thought I would love a doctor, but I love you," he professed.

His wife doubled the order and I fell back into the beautiful black hole of medicine, where love listens and learns and where science meets philosophy in an embrace with social graces that dares to touch another's flesh and lock eyes without threat.

Silly and stupid, I fell. "I really love you too," I replied. Time swirled in a whirlpool filled with numbers and chemicals. Receptors fell away from membranes, and new ones rose to the surface to embed readied. The telomeres pulled apart, and the focus was both head-on and spun in three dimensions to find depth, width, length. Then sound erupted and I just gasped and grabbed his hand and cried because I was tired of loving and losing. "Thanks for seeing me. Thanks for coming," he said, further piercing my heart to test its integrity too. I suddenly just wanted to take it all back and offer him a canyon climb. It would have been a lie, but one so American I could call it equally right.

All his friend's called him Tommy-boy. So like a British pop song with trumpets, Tommy-boy went home to die. He wanted to be home for Christmas to look at his decorations and the amber glow of his fine tree. "You might make it to Christmas," I offered, but that was a lie, as I regarded his blood pressure and him on room air for now. If he ate he would have just shy of ten days.

"I just have one question," he retorted. "Do you know where I can get the best fish and chips?"

"Pete's Fish and Chips," I professed. "Buy also the onion rings and get a lot of Pete's sauce. I don't know what's in it. Fancy ketchup but it's different. Also get a monster burger. Bring cash. They only take cash."

His wife resounded, "Oh my God, you two!"

We parted, I spewing out like a quasar.

Tommy-boy did not make it to Christmas. I do not even know if he got the fish and chips. Time for all of us never started up again in a way that a human could care. Gravity stayed poised at the newtons that define the moments before death when living is the heaviest. Tommy-boy became a black hole that stopped time and simultaneously stood in a perceived paradox of still being human without time to measure anything but a feeling left like a residue on paper after a story is written and read. He just stood and claimed love like an anchor and a goalpost. He just yielded and we marched time onward, being not the one dying this time.

And I fell right into the paradox peacefully with him and his wife.

Reference: https://www.nationalgeographic.com/science/article/black-holes

♥

The Bouquet

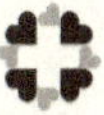

"Dr. Robey! Dr. Robey!" he yelled as I walked into the room. "Dr. Robey! Dr. Robey!" he leaped off his seat as if the name was rocket fuel and I was a cosmic kick.

I was smiling at his enthusiasm, and I looked closely at his face and his wife's face. His wife smiled so proudly and looked so pleased. Her eyes twinkled. His eyebrows rose and waggled in a chagrined and impish glee. They had candy and we were kids.

I was delighted but was not fully aware of why the fanfare. His wife read my slight misstep in comprehension. She percolated to tell me.

His wife unveiled, "Well . . . we figured out he could learn people's names again and . . . you're the only doctor he learned thus far. He couldn't wait to show you!"

"See. See here," he added as proof of his efforts. He pulled out of his breast pocket the most gorgeous three-by-five card I have ever seen, on which across the blue lines in black Sharpie was written, "Dr. Robey."

Four years earlier, a stroke had robbed his mind of words and left behind broken utterances and a stream of numbers as he fought to make meaningful dialogue. We struggled at first, but in time the string of numbers related to data he wanted to discuss. Blood sugars, blood pressures, electrolyte values, and kidney clearance.

"Like. Like Brian!" he announced, and flashed another three-by-five card.

"Yes. And . . ." she prompted.

"Ryan." He smiled and pulled out the corresponding card like a Vegas magician.

Brian and Ryan were their sons.

"And . . ." she beamed.

"Dr. Robey!" he belted and Charlie Chaplined his brow, waving the study aid with my name embossed.

I had achieved the awesome status of repopulating a mind. Me. My name. In a small and important stack. Me. My name.

My mind crashed into the mountain of flowers. This bouquet done this way was the best I ever could receive, and the embossed "Dr. Robey" three-by-five index card became the hallmark of love come full circle. I was going to have a name in this man's world. He surely was going to have place in my story doctoring. He had survived a stroke. And as thanks he saw to it that I survived the stroke too intact . . . with my name.

When the day closed, I grabbed a blank three-by-five card, like the thousands I had used to memorize so many facts, and wrote on it in black Sharpie . . . his name.

Ralph.

♥

Second Movement—Moonlight Sonata

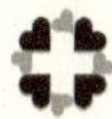

When I was six, I said for the first time I wanted to be a doctor. I played the hell out of a plastic stethoscope and a fake plastic medicine syringe with moving plunger. I was every stuffed animal's hero.

I started building my resume in eighth grade, and never did I relent.

I wanted into the fellowship of medicine.

Then she arrived in my office some twenty-two years later. White-haired and just nearing eighty, she was a mother of doctors and capable. I doctored her for over a decade, and she neared renal failure, to where we needed to meet up and talk about choices and goals and the growing statistic that in your nineties dialysis may lengthen life by six months but that length is hard-earned.

She flirted with death but retracted over and over again for a year away from the edge. The millimeters that signified imminent threat were her margin of error for so many puzzling months. I must have said goodbye four times, and every time that she made me a liar I was happy. We talked like I had a kettle on during office follow-ups. Then one day I was in the hospital rounding, and there she was admitted near a mile marker in the middle of no where, vibrantly alert but pathetically weak.

"What are you doing here?" I queried, knowing well it was the slow slide of inevitability.

"Waiting for this shit to close out," she scoffed.

Frankly, I loved her audacity and direct speak. She was ninety-one years old and pure and decisive, like a hot knife cutting cream cheese to smear onto life. She said everything straight and I laughed at the unlaughable moment her swearing created in her sterile and damning hospital room.

"I'm sorry I laughed. It's just miserable waiting. Are you comfortable? Do you want anything at all that I can order or get you?" I asked.

"I'm okay. I ate French toast," she replied like a kid on Sunday.

"You want a pound of bacon?" I offered with sincerity.

She laughed and felt satisfied at the idea.

"It's almost over," I reflected.

"Yeah, it is. I'm okay. I'm just waiting," she reassured.

"You know I love you. I can only say goodbye so easily because in my mind we will just meet up again and again like we have every time I keep saying goodbye. We just meet up again somewhere on a bench, visiting like we always have," I said, exposing my confidence.

"Oh, I know. I plan to save you a spot," she smiled. She was to be discharged on hospice to a nursing home.

We parted.

We waited.

A week later I got a potted orchid. She had sent one when I arranged her Covid vaccine in the days when getting one was challenging to thank me for early resourcefulness. "Another orchid, Dr. Robey," my medical assistant announced. I knew it was her. I knew why. But then the card was another level of astounding reflection. The card was handwritten, and in a waning blue cursive it said,

Dear Dr. Robey,

Thank you for caring for me all these long years. I will miss my appointment with you today and I'm sorry for that. I will however save you a stop on my bench up here.

Love,
Edith

She passed two days prior but had arranged for the flowers to arrive. I looked at my schedule and indeed she would have been my 10:15 a.m.

Edith,

May you always be the second movement in my sonata with medicine. The crushing blows of COVID nearly abducted my passion for doctoring. Those 2 brutal years threaten to eradicate a lifetime of wanting to be a physician and yet the orchid still blooms true.
I love medicine.
I loved being your doctor.

Love,
Dr. Robey

♥

Genetics

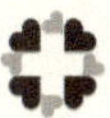

Two charts lay leaning in door racks, and the medical assistant flagged me down as I exited a third room laughing. The mood turned sober when I saw her face trying to interrupt gently.

"Mr. Silvestry said you said if he was ever around and needed you to stop in. He's here," she announced.

"Where is he?" I inquired, looking for doors eagerly yearning me in.

"In the waiting room . . . waiting," she clarified.

The day was piling like laundry, and I was about to try to freeze time. I opened the sacred dividing door to the crowded waiting room and loudly whispered my favoritism and waved Mr. Silvestry toward me, past the jealous faces. "Come. Come," I beckoned.

Mr. Silvestry got up quickly with a smile and tiptoed past a few perplexed onlookers. We merely stopped in the hallway to talk. As I shut the door after him, I looked him over, noticing he had lost twenty pounds. "You look . . . good," I gushed a bit, then touched his cheek as if I were assessing his composure. "How are you?" I asked.

His eyes welled up and he bit his lip and nodded with a lump in his throat. His beloved wife had passed three months earlier from endocarditis and septic shock, and he had agonized over the decision to withdraw care as she declined rapidly.

"What do you want to do?" the doctors had pressed.

"I want her to be well. I want her to wake up. I want her to go home. I want to sleep and never worry. I want to stop crying. I want to understand. I want something to blame. I want more time. I want to do the right thing. I want you to not ask me what I want," his mind raced. What he said, though, was, "I want to have her not suffer."

"I'm okay. I lost weight," he declared. I patted his belly lightly again as if I was studying his new package and assessing its fitness for journey.

"I had a question. You said I could come anytime to ask," he reminded me.

"Yes, of course. Ask me," I availed. I was prepared to relive the long, spiraling heartache. I shifted my weight to center my core.

"What happened to Eva," he began, "is it genetic? I mean, her brother and father both had kidney failure. Do I need to warn my kids?" he fretted.

Eva has been a nonsmoking vasculopath riddled with dozens of occlusions and in time kidney failure.

"Well, not exactly. She had horrible blood vessels so I would suggest your children take seriously not smoking, controlling weight, and addressing blood pressure and high cholesterol. But no. There is no true genetic factor I would test or treat directly," I surmised.

Mr. Silvestry was relieved. Then he exposed a deeper reality to me that sang like a harpy into the dark night. "I have six siblings. We have all outlived our spouses. What do you make of that?" he puzzled.

My skin prickled. I recalled tales of people who repeatedly married people who developed cancer later in life or spouses who had the same cancer where no one else who shared their environment did—or people drawn to people with multiple ironic meetings over a lifetime till they married. I saw Mr. Silvestry's holiday table lined with all the siblings and no guest married into the family. "Perhaps you all are destined not for grief but deep and needed love that is accentuated by loss," I hoped.

"I sure did love her. I was the last to lose a spouse—what do you think of that?" He shook his head.

I thought a million thoughts. I thought he looked tired and thin but fit enough. I thought he was processing his new reality okay. I thought he was admirable in trying to find meaningful use of tragic events for his children. I thought he was endearing and deep and human, digging deep into suffering and looking for something old and telling of existence. I thought what an incredible detail a string of spouseless siblings was. I thought my god, he is trying to make sure his children do not leave spouses heartbroken. How gorgeous is he who comes in one day to ask me a question like a gift?

"I'm so sorry for you and all your siblings. It is in our very genes and lifeline how we will journey. It was in yours to see me today and give me such a detail. Your children are half you and half your wife. Your children and wife, though, have all your heart, so chances are they will always be well-loved. Try not to worry. Be smart but don't linger too long in fear. Our fates should not sacrifice our days and freeze our living," I pondered.

"Thank you for seeing me. You said if I ever was around to stop in. Thank you," he cherished.

"Of course. I stopped Time, and Time gave me and others something to think on. Love is powerful medicine. Nothing is more human. Nothing more basic in our genes. "Love is genetic and primordial," I loved him back.

♥

Accounting

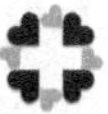

She struck me immediately.

I think it was the way she rose or shook my hand and smiled with certainty. I knew she was a direct person and comfortable being such.

"What did you do in your past life?" I inquired.

"Well," she laughed, "I was a housewife, but when the girls got to college, well," she contemplated, "we needed the money, so I went to work as an accountant."

I love accountants. They see little details like a nephrologist does.

She was new to my practice, and I was just getting to know her numbers and needs. She was easy to make laugh and smile despite the myriad medical issues she navigated.

"You know," she added to the column, "my husband was on dialysis for five years."

Speaking in the past tense with a tone of authority and love, I knew three things: she was a woman of experience, she was a woman of accountability, and she was a woman still grieving this loss. I inquired a bit further. "Oh," I started in, "why was he on dialysis?"

She told a tale of early heart attacks and three bypass surgeries and a dozen stents even before his eventual renal failure. Upon the hour of his renal expiration, she told of a tale involving another nephrologist far away. "And that nephrologist tried to talk him out of dialysis when he was failing," she saddened.

I added across the grid and found myself a bit short too with his odds and his potential. "Well," I confessed, "I think he might have been at risk for many things given his severe heart disease, to be honest. As you know, dialysis is a marathon of sorts, and a gentleman with such miserable heart issues could have really been taxed by dialysis."

She acquiesced and saw perhaps the past nephrologist's agenda in a new, more caring light. She nodded and forgave him for being "discouraging."

"How did he pass away?" I investigated upon seeing a blank box in another row.

"Would you believe it, pancreatic cancer?" she exclaimed.

Apparently, her husband Russell was having some vague stomach pains. They found pancreatic cancer in the later stages, and he swiftly decided to pursue no treatment and to withdraw from dialysis. It was hard to weigh in after so much time, but in retrospect my boldest reflection to her was that we should be thankful for renal failure since then a stopping point could be declared in the face of certain suffering and impasse. "He got actually a choice to stop dialysis and succumb gently to the truth of all things converging," I summed.

She agreed.

"For two weeks after he was off dialysis, our daughters came home to help me care for him. These two daughters were so amazing and did things no daughter should ever have to do for their father, but he thanked them every day. He would say 'Thank you so much' to each so gently," she shared.

I saw Russell, thin and frail, humbling himself to be bathed and carried by his grown daughters. I saw him carefully tell them thank you and then I saw him fade down a river of uremia and sleep.

She agreed.

The column was adding up so sweetly and then she added a row I truly felt blessed to share as I kept her in the office past the point of my own value as a nephrologist and contribution medically. "My husband was a man who would give me fresh flowers each month," she teared up. "Toward the end about two weeks before he was diagnosed with pancreatic cancer he started bringing me fresh flowers . . . after each dialysis. Three times a week he would bring them home . . . Monday, Wednesday, Friday," she conjured. The aroma and sight of arrays of fresh flowers filled my office as she described them. "I think he knew," she sighed. "I got so many bouquets. He would say to me, 'You're so beautiful.'"

I agreed. She was bathed in perfumes as she spoke and looked in love and lovely.

"Ma'am," I shared, "there are many selfish reasons I have kept you here, but please know these last have been the most lovely. I often must tell patients their kidneys are failing and that they must now entertain dialysis 'three times a week.' It is hard to hear that you must commit to a treatment 'three times a week' to stay alive, but when you created this image of fresh flowers from your lover three times a week—Monday, Wednesday, Friday—who could refuse such a life extended? I thank you for your story."

She agreed.

"I'm so happy you are here. I write stories. I usually write of my patients and my time with them. I am most sad I did not know Russell. Could I, may I ask, could I write of him anyway?" I hoped.

She smiled wide and delighted. The columns were added up in the black. "Please do! We would love that," she agreed.

And here is, thus, the math of the moment. Fresh flowers every month for 37 years + 3 bypass surgeries + 12 stents + 5 years on dialysis + fresh flowers three times a week for 2 weeks + 2 daughters + 1 cancer to best, uremic and peaceful, + 1 direct and loving wife = a life robust and revisited and 1 story to tell.

♥

One Tour

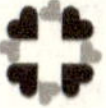

In the concourse of a day, the highway of a week, the six-lane freeway of a month in which a call weekend falls and lines up fourteen days working in a row, I sit and stand and buckle like a lumberjack log-walking on the river, logs rolling.

Day 1, Room 2:

"I wish you weren't my doctor," he stung, then soothed with clarification, "so we could be neighbors and speak of everything else on any day."

Day 1, Room 3:

He had arrived to our attention after doctors looking for a cause for constipation incidentally found "the largest aneurysm" many had ever recalled seeing. At 9.3 cm, the aortic aneurysms heralded an alarm. He stood to die not of the prostate cancer they treated years ago but the sudden rupture of his vasculature, exsanguinating in an instant. Everyone marveled at how curious it was for complaints of constipation to prompt a lifesaving CT scan. He was hospitalized immediately for surgery. That hospitalization was rather uneventful and he came to my office as a post-hospitalization follow-up given findings then of renal impairment. I had never met him before as another nephrologist had seen him while he was in the hospital.

"Have you ever seen a kidney doctor before this hospitalization?" I sought to establish.

He was calmly dressed in a clean t-shirt and creased shorts. I found him fit and was surprised how unscathed he was by the near-death drama. His body was stented along the main aorta and stented into both renal arteries. He hands were folded in his lap. He seemed peacefully accepting.

"That's an interesting question," he began. The whirlwind threw us back in time, and I saw him dazzled by the urgency but walking on his own accord into hospital admission. He was rushed to this test, rushed to that room, rushed back, rushed to sign, rushed to another room, rushed back to his room, rushed to eat, proven stable, rushed home "to follow up," rushed to call, then suddenly stopped on the making of an available appointment with the first nephrologist that could see him.

"I was supposed to see this other nephrologist after the stents, but he was booked so I was to see this other doctor, but he said no because it was professional courtesy for the first to see me so he refused, so I just waited to see you as you opened this spot, which landed me exactly here," he weaved.

My heart smiled with pleasure as the universe sent me a gift.

"Well, I must say you are rather calm despite the amazing journey you've had, finding fortuitously such a startling-sized aneurysm and being whisked away to fix it. You could've just died one day abruptly," I reflected.

He chuckled. "So I have been told by many."

"Furthermore, all this tossing about not having a catcher for your kidney worries must have made for mixed feelings and frustration or at least this anticlimactic moment," I continued.

He smiled and tilted his head and nodded.

"I am amazed by your composure, which I feel is part ignorance, part denial, part shock, part sensibility, part faith, part charm," I dared.

He was intrigued.

"But," I exclaimed, "I shall promise to reward you and thank you!"

He adjusted in his seat and readied anxiously to see how possibly he would come out ahead.

We spoke of all medications, all medical problems, all matters still at hand, all labs, all emotions, all crazed ideas, and in the end, "I really will enjoy your company for here on out, my lucky friend! I find your happenstance to my exam room a pleasant gift. I hope you do too."

He searched his mind for the title of a book that the moment reminded him of. "Argh. You'd think I would recall! It was one I taught from for decades," he chagrined.

"Oh? You were a teacher?" I asked.

"Yeah, I taught English. Oh, what was that book?" he belabored.

I was typing and so without looking I offered, "*The Alchemist*?" He enthusiastically replied, "Yes! That's the one. The Universe conspires!"

"Indeed, it does," I connected. Being a reader, I had won him completely.

Day 5, phone encounter:

"Thank you for coming by that day when my mother ran into you. My father was so surprised to see you visit. When you left he told everyone he thought you liked him!" the junior shared, laughing at the thought of admiration on my part toward his father.

"But I do. He's a fine friend," I confirmed, genuinely intrigued by the retired criminal detective. "One of the first times we met up he profiled me but was most surprised by the experience of being profiled himself by me!"

Day 13, online email:

"No offense. I prefer a male doctor. Can you refill my metoprolol?" the queued inquiry read.

I replied, "Not a problem. You must seek who you feel connected to best. I have refilled the medication. Further replies and assistance will be from your new physician," I closed.

Day 14, email from team member:

"I have spoken to Mr. Edwards' daughter. She says he is not eating off and on and not speaking off and on. She said she spoke to you earlier this week and he's 'about the same really,' but I thought I would tell you because something in her voice seemed to need to speak to you again." —Candice

Candice was a dietitian who never steered me wrong, so I obeyed her intuition and dialed the daughter. It was 9:08 a.m. Meanwhile, my 9:00 a.m. patient finally was roomed and waiting.

"Hello?" Rose answered.

"Hello, Rose. It's Dr. Robey. Candice emailed me and told me you two spoke. Something made her feel I should call you, though I realize he hasn't changed since we last spoke. What else is happening?" I invited.

She was quiet, then sighed and started. "He's the same. I guess . . ." She hesitated, then the words rolled forward swiftly. "I don't know what to do. I'm . . ." She paused and inhaled. "I'm getting married and he was supposed to go to respite care, but truly, Dr. Robey I am so conflicted. My constant tending is all that keeps this barely afloat, and I feel like if he goes to respite . . ." She stopped.

"The ship will sink," I declared.

"Yes. It will totally sink," she owned.

"When is the wedding?" I sought to clarify.

"In ten days," she outlined.

"Then what after? Are you home again or planning a trip?" I pursued.

"We had planned a honeymoon," she shamed.

"Well, listen," I offered. "This is a wonderful and amazing thing. Do not deny yourself this joy. Life is brutal; it seems to make the passing of your father collide with this joy, but perhaps I can do three things."

She listened.

"First, your father has been dying for eight months. He has drifted slowly. This is not a new revelation, and so do not feel you are giving up or are willing its end. Secondly, it is not your burden to bear this alone or singularly in life's balance. I watched as you played out the last months as you could to honor your needs and love, but truly I could have evoked martial law at any time to say he is not a dialysis candidate and should stop and be made comfortable. I will do this now. Finally, sometimes it is the case that a great day is chosen for an equally bad day or event to fall around to help one emotion counter another. Do you understand? It may be that you having an amazing wedding and new life helps you move on against this impending loss." I had attempted to rearrange the landscape.

She was ripe with sleepless nights and raw thought. "I have been thinking," she confessed, "since our last conversation. I have been thinking so hard. I just . . ." she stammered.

"You are a great daughter. Let me help you. Rest your trust in that I have cared for and of your father for a long time. I mean him no harm and can help you both. You think about what I'm saying. I recommend he stops dialysis and enrolls in hospice today. You may tell anyone who asks that I medically see the need. They should not blame you nor see this as an act of convenience. I shall call you at 2 p.m. today," I ended, and she agreed to think on things.

The 9 a.m. patient waited patiently, aware what waiting meant they did so for someone else. My patients are conditioned to save space knowing they may cycle through as the one in need.

Day 14, 9:22 a.m.

"I'm sorry I am late," I apologized, rushing in.

"It's completely okay. I am retired," she laughed at her awesome luck.

"Nevertheless, I never assume nor should you just give your time away without good cause and sincere apologies," I attested. She nodded, accepting both knowing the practice style I gave and all received by test of time.

Day 14, phone encounter, 2:03 p.m.:

"Hello?" Rose answered.

"Hello. It is Dr. Robey. Have you had a chance to speak to your fiancé and family?" I followed up.

"Yes. I have. We decided that your advice is very appropriate," she bowed to admit.

I reached through the phone and took her chin and raised it up and looked her in the eyes. "It is okay. I will arrange everything. They will contact you today."

"Thank you, Dr. Robey," she relieved.

"Thank you, Rose. Your father is very lucky and will be happily at your wedding in spirit. Please look at it like that," I encouraged. "Do you need me to call anyone else?" I offered, sensing her guard.

"Yes. Would you? Can you call my brother?" she asked shyly.

"Of course. I shall do so now," I closed.

I dialed several times, finally leaving a message. The 2:15 p.m. patient roomed. I vowed to try again at 4:00.

Day 14, phone encounter, 6:04 p.m. on the way home:

"Hello?" the phone picked up.

"Michael Edwards?" I asked by way of timely intrusive assumptions.

"This is him," he said leerily.

I apologized for the abruptness of meeting but also the delay well past 4 p.m. and launched into an effort to clarify the design for his father.

"I want to thank you for calling and for telling Rose she could have a life. She's been so dedicated but these last months just seem so draining," he thanked.

Given his already timely agreeance and my mounting piles of obligations, we ended the call in minutes. He did not need the call but his sister needed to know she was not the instrument by her need or design. I could quickly deliver that objectivity and unburden her narrative.

Then . . . I drove my car into the garage and sat in the quiet space to take inventory of a long tour of sorting and stabilizing problems daily for fourteen straight days. People collided and circled in the forever arena ongoing, and the full weight of sonder sat beside me. I opened the car door and exited the welcomed solitude and invited the noises of my own personal universe, unfolding among the celestial planets I called my own.

♥

"Send Help."

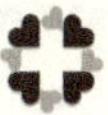

He drove himself to my office. When he arrived, he casually waited in the room, and when I entered he rose and greeted me. He had maintained the weight he had lost so expeditiously after one read of *The Obesity Code*. When he finished the read, he handed the book over and told me to give it to someone else. That afternoon, I promptly reissued it.

I casually greeted him back and went about my business of organizing his data points.

"I passed out the other day," he confessed.

"Oh?" I paused. "Then what happened?"

He shifted ever so slightly in his chair and then resumed a storyline midway. "Well, I pulled over into the turning lane," he continued.

To that I turned fully to look at him, puzzled by his details, disoriented by the geography laid out.

"You were driving?" I queried.

"Yeah, so I pulled over into the turning lane," he reiterated.

"You were driving and pulled over into the left-hand turning lane?" I clarified.

He continued to build the disbelief. "I came to in the turning lane, then turned and then I passed out again so I pulled over but came to." He motioned with his hands on an imaginary steering wheel.

Like a parrot I repeated, "You were passing out so you pulled into the left turning lane, came to, and then turned left and was passing out again so you pulled over and came to?"

"Yeah," he exacted.

I fell dumbfounded and dared to ask, "Then what? Did you call 911 and go to the hospital?"

"No," he plainly spoke. "I came to so I went home."

It had been a week since his events, and he denied any prodrome other than the slow awareness of losing consciousness. He had no current symptoms, and it being a routine appointment, I had labs around the time of the event and all was well.

"Listen to me," I cautioned, "if you have any issues at all again, you must call 911."

He looked at me but did not hear me at all and felt the superficial breeze of my caution touching treetops in a dense forest. I rolled over in my stool and lightly touched his arm. "Listen. To. Me," I heralded. "Sometimes we are given three warnings. You in the turning lane, you pulling over. That is two warnings and the third will be your last. When that happens, despite your wish for other things to be the case, you must call 911. I would send you now to the hospital, but I have no cause and you won't go anyway. But hear me now. *If* you have another anything, you must call 911."

He looked at me with dewy eyes and nodded hypnotically. My melodrama scared him, and I took my time turning my back to him, keeping my head and eyes transfixed on him like a ballerina spotting.

That night he lay in bed, awoken by chest pain. Feeling it a bout of reflux, he turned over and met his wife awake. "What's wrong?" she asked. He brushed it off, saying at first, "It's nothing, just some . . ." but trailed off. He then told his wife to call 911, and off they were, taken to a quick evaluation and an even more rapid and frightfully eventful trip to the CATH lab. He had two stents placed. I called him the next morning after hearing of the admission.

"Mr. Steward," I said.

"I know that voice," he replied.

"Mr. Steward," I repeated in a tone of tsk-tsk and joy.

He laughed and confessed, "I was going to roll over and go back to bed after I reassured my wife, but then I heard your voice say, 'Go now,' and I switched and told her to call 911. It felt pretty theatrical until, well, it wasn't. They say I will be okay."

I laughed at the image of my haunting voice. I appreciated that he had taken the good measure to heed it. "Otherwise," I said, "I would have come to kill you myself for not listening."

The next day he was discharged and enrolled in outpatient cardiac rehab. On the third week while on the treadmill, he had a brief bradycardic episode and felt woozy. He stopped and again contemplated something off-world and asked the therapist to call 911.

"I heard your voice again," he later claimed, and it said again, 'Go now,' so I went.

I laughed at his unusual luck and my newfound ability to haunt the living. He had an in-stent blockage, and a stent was placed to stabilize him.

Randomly one morning, he arrived on my office schedule one month earlier than expected.

"I was just talking about you to another man who can't seem to remember to drink enough water but says he is trying better as he hears my voice lecturing him constantly," I laughed.

He laughed at the thought of my multiple hauntings but his face grew sad to miss out. "I'm here to say goodbye," he shared sorrowfully. "We are moving in the next week to Missouri."

"Oh? That is so sad to hear but exciting too," I exclaimed, knowing I would miss his visits to remind me of things that happenstance.

I asked why Missouri and if they had found a house. He smiled knowing I would ask for more details. "Well, after the first near-miss

I asked my wife where she wanted to die and she said near her kids in Missouri. I was so tired for so long that it seemed that I just did not get around to finding a house. I found one recently. It's 150 years old and the real deal. A beautiful Victorian style actually and we love it." He showed me photos, so very proud of the woodwork. I thought the house was such an extension of how long he aspired to live timelessly and now with wiser caution too.

He thanked me, of course, and said that even the day before he had heard my voice. "I was fixing a wire up in the ceiling and would need a twelve-foot ladder. I heard you say, 'Act eighty, not thirty,' and I called my son to come do it." I laughed at the third haunting and hugged him long.

"Thank you again for saving me," he hugged back.

"It is amazing how we save each other," I countered.

♥

The Little Things

She pulled a tray over and opened a few things, organizing the silverware and cutting the chicken. With the fork and knife already in her hands, she scooped a bit of mashed potatoes and forked the chicken, adding a slither of sundried tomato to the heap and a shriveled spinach leaf in a lovely, picturesque, mouthwatering bite.

He was masked and unconscious. Someone had forgotten to change the dietary order and someone had delivered the tray anyway to the otherwise isolated room. He would never eat it but poising him on the brink of a morsel so designed seemed to affirm he was human awaiting a bite of living.

The TV was playing a silly show, and so she turned it to fireworks and left the fork of food so nicely layered on the edge of the plate.

He had lingered for twenty-one days, not one visitor awaiting a fiduciary, and so she left him to linger in a room safe and cool as the outdoors remained a hot box of 102 degrees.

He might have been Republican or Democrat. He might have never exercised a vote or cared too much about a neighborhood. He might have loved the girl next door or the guy from work but never did he have children. He might have said goodbye to the ones he knew years ago and waited quietly in God's waiting room just to test all of us with how kind we might be to such a lesser seen creature.

He just waited for any person to come and engage him. He just languished to test anyone's awareness of another. He was flatly "just." He just laid around, being a must to no one in particular, but here, she treated him properly.

"Happy 4th of July," she whispered and left the room.

♥

One Chair

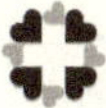

I remember two chairs facing south against a white wall facing me, with me on the left and a cabinet behind my right shoulder. The exam table faced north. The door was in the right north corner. I remember that she was always in the chair by the door and he was in the chair in the corner because he rested his head against where the walls met, and it looked cozy. I remember I was always tired, and nestling a head wedged where two walls met looked so great I was envious. I remember because every visit for years, I could tell if they were not in the same cozy room where I met them first and last. Today we were in the room I see in my mind, but she was alone sitting in "her chair." "His chair" was empty.

I blew in and turned to see his chair empty and joked, "Where's your husband? Off doing your bidding?"

She said he was not feeling well.

I apologized, and we rifled through things together, but simultaneously I explored, "What's wrong with Bill?"

Bill had survived Stage 3 melanoma with reoccurrence. For eight years he was disease-free. He had beaten the odds and had been given the cavalier clean bill of health last fall that said they were done with serial imaging.

Bill had started having a pain in his right upper quadrant just before a much-awaited cruise was planned to begin a month earlier. He did a litany of things and eventually they requested a CT scan "given his history."

We have heard this story, so we knew that his fate turned and the scan showed a mass on the liver and enlarged lymph nodes and another mass in the lung. We have heard this story because we are doctors. Yet . . .

She composed herself briefly, then got on the exam table and sobbed in between my exam.

"So, they said for us to go on our cruise," she cried. "They said they would have everything ready for us when we returned." She described every day of the cruise. "I try to believe the things people say about God, the things I say about God. I try to smile. What will I do without my husband?" They returned to port and then to a reality of time running out. She cried a river, and I wadded my paddle boat over.

"Move over," I said, and she made way for me and we sat shoulder to shoulder on the exam table looking at the two empty chairs. We could've been on a ledge overlooking the city. Her warmth was evident, and I could smell her lotions and salty tears. The horizon was ours to describe.

I exhaled.

"Listen to my story," I started. "Long ago I cared for a woman. She sat in that chair." I pointed to the very chair she had sat in. "I never met her husband. They were deeply in love because she spoke of him often. One day she came in and told me he had Stage 4 lung cancer. At first he was okay, then good, then again okay, then suddenly one day she came in and told me and he had turned for the worse and died. She fell into a deep depression. For a year I dragged her out. She hated God. She broke with him and felt hateful of life. She ate ice cream every day and that is all she could do."

She listened.

"There is nothing I can tell you that you have not heard except that I hear past many things and hope I can start a conversation that saves you when . . . when the journey ends. He has Stage 4 melanoma and there are new medicines that they are trying. We will hope and we savor each day, but let me make sure that when the journey is over you are okay to weather that storm too."

She seemed to understand the beacon I placed far into the future. It shined as a post far off to reach for. It gave her anchor and assurance. Today was today. Tomorrow was certain in other ways. Battling today should not negate every tomorrow. There would be ice cream or some small token that drags us forward. Life mandates this truth.

I paddled away and made an appointment for six months. I offered one sooner, should she have the need.

"A lot can happen in six months," she worried.

"Time is like a crumpled piece of paper. Time touches many edges, and thus things that have happened or will happen are already upon us. I am here. Just reach out. But do not fear time and circumstance. We are merely passing through and around it. We are readying ourselves for fights while fighting. I am here," I assured her. "Meet me at that equinox and I will hear your tale. Meet me and let us see what we are to do next."

She kept her appointments and updated me through the hellfire of trying. Oddly and amazingly, he survived well past the six months they were given and went on two more cruises, and in time she was faced with his passing. But his presence remained in my appointments with her in the one chair we left open. In that design is how we all see each day through to the next.

♥

Not a Fiber

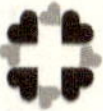

In December, in the first year of the Covid pandemic, we met for the second time and he said yet again, "I'm only here because a friend said I should meet you." He told me about his life over ninety-two years, and eventually he shared that his children had recently moved back in to help him manage his blind, demented wife. "I want her home with me, and they are making it possible." He described the landscape of his most current chapter that I was invited to only via "a friend."

We gathered again today in April via telephone only.

"Do you have an iPhone?" I inquired, thinking I could interface with his . . . face.

"A what?" he puzzled. "I have just a landline," he justified, slightly annoyed by the burden of this diligence to meet with me.

I affirmed, "That will do just fine."

We ran the gauntlet. He was doing well. No cough, chest pain, shortness of breath, fever, chills, or diarrhea. His laboratory values were "steady Freddy," he confirmed. Then he ended with, "So my wife passed last week. I told you about her being ill."

I opened the floor for him to speak, and so the tale goes . . .

"She died peacefully at home. She was by my side. Then came the strangest thing. They would not let us gather at the cemetery for a funeral. Just the gravediggers were there. Just the gravedigger, you know," he stammered.

I could feel the quiver of his voice unsteadied in a rocky walk in a spacey universe, so I grabbed hold of him to ground us and invited, "Walk me through this. Tell me again what happened."

"Well, see. They took her body away, then called me. They asked if I wanted to delay the funeral, and I just couldn't having been with her for some seventy years. Then how my kids did these things the last year, like they did to just wait on this peace for her and us so . . . I waited at home and told them to go ahead and bury her. I just sat at home trying to think on her and thank the gravediggers for their time in my mind quietly," he steadied.

Then I quivered as part transference and part my own reaction to the echo of "the gravediggers, the gravediggers, the gravediggers" placing her ashes in a holy hole in the ground at the military cemetery.

"I was military. World War II. Never not been to a funeral," he swore. Then, "I cleaned the patio today," he sighed. "Me and my children. They've been such a blessing. I really love them here with me."

"What a beautiful thing to have right now during such science-fictional times. I am so sorry for your loss, and then these details that I can only say prove you haven't a selfish fiber in your soul. Most people don't know what to choose in extreme moments. You, however, I have seen, and with this last act of potentially unresolved and unsatisfying love I see that you have not one fiber of selfishness. Astonishingly, these times unearth the depths of a person, revealing valor such as yours," I marveled.

"Thank you. I have very good friends too," he smiled. "One recommended I see you, and I guess I needed to for many reasons," he laughed.

"I needed you too," I owned.

When we could not gather at a funeral, we were tested, and some of us stood to learn a lot from just an old man checking in, telling a tale to a lover of stories.

♥

The Labyrinth Unraveling

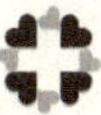

"Your mother put the top to the blender somewhere." My husband was casting blame as he banged through a dozen cabinets, searching.

"Your mother," I tossed.

"Your mother," he rallied.

"Your. Mother," I hustled, swung, and the phrase went out of bounds.

Love/15

The running joke was our mothers would invariably relocate items upon visiting intentionally to thwart us. If something went missing it did so with a common rationale: "Your mother . . ."

"Your mother moved the big red pot," I claimed once as I scoured the pantry.

"Your mother lost our wine opener," he declared most weekends, as he pushed around cutlery.

"Your mother likely threw out the cold brew top," I declared as I dug through the trash as if his mother drank cold brew at all.

One day, my husband's mother came to visit. Compared to two years ago, her memory was fading fast. Within minutes, she would repeat a story or detail. She would begin a long novel and forget the plot and characters. I studied her to see if I could understand what new idea would stay and what ideas would fly fast away. It turned out that events told with complex happenings would remain long enough to sink like small rocks into the soft gray matter of her mind. Emotional details became the sticky parts of events that her mind could adhere to. The hockey game where we ate pulled pork sandwiches and she shared her chips with me, the three-mile loop we walked around the nearby resort where horses neighed, or the trip with growing grandkids to Junipine among the fall colors and smell of pine burning remained, but the random details unhooked to any important happenings like the gate code or the date of her flight home would flutter away. She would repeat herself, so I in kind repeated myself too.

The first time would be, "There's a blue afghan that I'll mail home." To which I would reply, "Oh? Would you like me to do that for you?"

The second time would be, "There's a blue afghan that I'll mail home," which was met with initially silence as I took in what was to happen for her or me next. I did not mind hearing her thoughts again, considering it was just conversation; I felt happy to have it with her. Yet, I could not bring myself to repeat my reply. To her I was just rudely quiet and unengagingly discourteous. To her first and only reality, I seemed to not care.

"Mom," I asked, "do you feel badly if we tell you that you have said something before?"

She pushed her well-earned pride aside.

"I guess I do a little," she admitted. "Did I tell you about the afghan before?"

"Yeah," I shrugged. "But Mom," I continued, "do you . . . do you get to feeling like . . . like not talking because you'll be foolish—appearing that you're repeating yourself?"

"Sometimes," she considered, "I think that being quiet is . . . safer," she divulged.

My heart ached as I saw her alone and unsure as to what thoughts she had shared and why comments from her had no reactions so often these days. I felt her fading from a place within conversation.

My heart ached to feel her growing closed off in the confines of only a safe, small, habitual world.

Mom walked into the kitchen and began to wash the dishes, feeling useful hiding behind the hot water and soap suds. She dried each plate thoughtfully and then walked around the kitchen trying to decide where the dishes belonged. I saw her doubtful and discouraged by forgetfulness and offered lovingly, "Oh, Mom, just place them anywhere."

"They need a place so I can remember where to put them," she chuckled.

I laughed with her for the hundredth time as we ran the same engagement over dishes "anywhere" and dishes "needing a place" and experienced together how the labyrinth unravels.

"I should mail the blue afghan," she fretted, matching the plates as a sign they belonged together, now clean, to those waiting to be used. It dawned on me some strategy after all to keep her here with me in conversation.

"Oh? Tell me again where you got that afghan," and the conversation continued to flow even with new angles and constant adoration.

♥

Ethics Committee

"They are killing me here. They are trying to kill me," Agnes cried out. She sat still with the bloodlines pumping her blood through the dialysis filter. "Help. They are killing me here."

Agnes looked around the room at the busy technicians and other patients. They seemed calm and orderly. "Why would people be so calm in a place where they kill people?" Agnes wondered. "Help," she quietly muttered as a nurse walked by.

Agnes's sitter sat watching television. She grew deaf to Agnes's cries as did everyone in the room.

Agnes had returned from her six-month stay in Washington. She returned to her unit in Arizona and to her station to dialyze. It was never Monday then Tuesday then Wednesday then Thursday then Friday then Saturday then Sunday. It was sometimes meatloaf day but mostly it was just a day and randomly it seemed her family would take her to this place.

"They are trying to kill me here," she would repeatedly say almost unaware of her words as she looked around.

"Agnes, it's all okay. We are almost done with your treatment," the nurse called out without even making eye contact.

"They are almost ready to kill me," Agnes said. Agnes would then tear up and then suddenly forget why she was crying.

We all sat in the conference room and readied ourselves for the meeting. Agnes's daughter was coming in to meet and reestablish care. Prior to Agnes leaving Washington, an Ethics Committee was convening to help determine the choices made by Agnes's family. Agnes's husband was still adamant about keeping her alive, and the daughters facilitated her sitters and transportation to the dialysis units.

"Welcome back, Mrs. Edwards," I greeted Agnes's eldest daughter. She was a kind lady with a slight drawl. She ended sentences with an agreeable "all right." I didn't feel any pretense or personal agenda. She seemed earnest and loving. "How was your mother's time in Washington?"

Mrs. Edwards shook my hand and sat. "Thank you. It was good. She did all right."

"Mrs. Edwards," I dove in, "your mother to me is no different than she was when she left. She still is very disoriented when she comes here. I dialyze demented patients at times. That doesn't concern me except that in her disorientation she has a moment of true fear and I believe feels we are trying to kill her. I can only imagine what that feels like for three and a half hours, three times a week. How is your mother at home otherwise?" I probed.

"She's fine. She just piddles around. She watches television and often cooks meals," her daughter testified.

"I see. Well I was told the Ethics Committee was still convening to evaluate her continued dialysis in Washington. Do you and your family feel she should continue dialysis?" I asked very directly.

"For now I think yes," she replied calmly.

"Well, as I have said she hadn't changed much from when she was here before. She was crying out then and the sitter would redirect and distract her. If, as her medical power of attorney you want to continue dialysis I will not refuse her, but please consider what I have said. For those moments she is here I think she may at times truly feel the terror of pending death repeatedly. It is a horrible thought to fathom," I insisted.

The weeks passed. The new sitter seemed frustrated caring for Agnes and having to remind her constantly she was "safe" and "no one was trying to kill her." Agnes became like a plant, ushered to and from dialysis.

"I think the sitter is not as nice as the prior one," my clinic nurse observed. "She seems to yell at Agnes."

Then one day a six-page summary of the convened Ethics Committee was forwarded to me. I did not read it. The verdict summary on the last page was that Agnes needed to withdraw from dialysis. I was not exactly sure by what authority.

Mrs. Edwards reached out to me.

"Hello, Mrs. Edwards. I received a very detailed summary from the Ethics Committee in Washington concerning your mother. I understand she is withdrawing from dialysis. Are you and your family okay with this?" I inquired. I did not tell her I had not read the "report." Mrs. Edwards sighed a draw and replied, "Well yes, it's all right. They found a form she filled out in 1996 that said she didn't want any aggressive care so I guess it's all right."

"Mrs. Edwards," I ventured, "you know it doesn't take a six-page summary to tell you why it's all right to stop dialysis. I see what you and your sister have tried to do for your father. It is hard to know what to do when someone seems still mostly there. I know it feels wrong to not just keep going. I know it feels wrong to suddenly stop something that hasn't changed in a year. I know it seems like a small thing to hire sitters and bring her to the unit three times a week. I know you deserve someone to tell you what to do. I want you to know I understand and that what matters most is what I have told you has been your mother's perception for some time now. In those hours and moments on dialysis your mother has suffered repeatedly the worst fears a person can have. She has felt the imminent dread of near death. She cannot escape this except to be allowed to stay at home and just piddle and make do. Don't do any more dialysis simply because she would have more moments of joy. Dialysis is meant to stave off death but not to repeatedly invite the fear of death."

I desperately wanted Mrs. Edwards to be the source of humane choices, not a committee's interpretation and imposition. "I see what you and your sister have tried to do. I know you tried to choose the lesser wrong or the most right. It's time to let nature release her from her mind's hell," I conveyed.

Mrs. Edwards was crying now. She had placed me on speakerphone, and Agnes's husband spoke up. "Dr. Robey, we will do just that. We will let her go. Today was her last treatment. We just decided ourselves."

I hung up the phone wishing them well and promising to arrange hospice for them. Agnes's dialysis chair would be reassigned to another person looking for more time and an honest fight against dying. Her cries would no longer be heard in the unit. She would never again fear the imminence of her death, being allowed instead to die. The family was going to be released from a cold verdict. The committee would merely stand as a launching pad. The six detailed pages that wove the logistic arguments to include old papers signed in vague ways would never inflate as the impetus that took control away from those left behind. The committee welcomed the family to the edge of deciding, and the family decided for themselves.

We must help families decide and to help them be okay with decisions they make long after a committee convenes. There will never be enough pages to summarize to the heart a defense against guilt. The rapport medicine fights to retain will strain under text and bullet points. It is a balance between all the ethical pillars in medicine including a bit of paternalism to release a person and their loved ones from the chains of what we can do.

♥

At the Stroke of Dependence, Half an Hour Past Independence

Carey came into my office every three to four months for ten years. "Are you married?" I initially asked.

Carey laughed and replied, "Well, I have this guy I've been going with for forty years now."

Her boyfriend was over ten years her senior. Carey was eighty when I met her. Her boyfriend had just turned 102.

Today Carey came into the office after two strokes with her daughter in the lead. I had never met her daughter because I had never needed to meet her. Today Carey was escorted by her daughter because after the stroke Carey "veers left when she walks, can't drive, is forgetful, and is flustered by frustration."

"Okay, up on the exam table," I directed Carey. "You know it's my physical fitness test." Long ago my attending in training told me if a patient could not mount or dismount the exam table it was an immediate indication for poor long-term prognosis. He would go so far as to dare not offer dialysis to the patient because long-term they "would fail anyway." With all the seriousness of an Olympic judge, I watched.

Carey walked over to the exam table and approached it on the left, then rethought and came instead from the right. It took her five steps to get up and turn around, and she sat up without aid.

Mount: 9.6

I examined her and then, while leaving her up there with me close by, I spoke to Carey.

"Well, your labs say your insides are fine, but you look so dejected. I'm afraid long before you die of illness you will die of devaluation of self," I declared.

Carey laughed and her smile was crooked on the right.

"I'm so disgusted," she began. "They want to all do stuff for me and tell me what to do and I'm so disgusted!" Her words slurred a bit. She never drooled.

Carey recanted a long list of things she couldn't do. She couldn't drive. She couldn't go anywhere alone. She couldn't shop. She couldn't pay bills. She couldn't speak at times.

"I see. You are having a tremendous amount of change and have no self-worth left. You know what the best way to handle this is?" I offered.

Carey sat forward, eager to fix her disheartened existence. Her torso was straight, and she didn't slouch or lean.

"To fix this we must be very strong and do something near impossible," I began.

Carey folded forward with firm flexion of her rectus and maintained herself on the exam table steadily. I noted her persistently strong tone and core balance.

"We must revalue ourselves," I declared, then paused. The words flirted with ridiculous. I continued, "We must take a kind of inventory and reassess our own metric to which we measure our worth of existence," I said, threatening the norm.

Carey chuckled.

"I'm serious," I contended. "Listen, dead is dead. Death will come for you. Death is already on the books for us all. Death waits already. When death comes the door closes and you are gone. Right now, you are alive. We are having a conversation and I am fully here feeling engaged. You are alive and engaged. Thus, you have value to me, your daughter, your family, your boyfriend. You exist and thus are of value. You need help. Take it. I know you value independence and value yourself only if you are independent, but you need to renegotiate the terms of your existence and realize what makes us of value is being capable of accepting new valuations and enjoying life till death comes. Your family wants you safe and well and happy. You must make safe choices, stay well, and learn to be happy again before you go forever and leave us all sad. Being here is an achievement, and staying to stay engaged is of value," I said, serenading her soul with gowns of diamond breath and shoes of eager talks.

Carey's eye contact never wavered, and her comprehension was intact.

Showmanship: 10.0

Carey rose to dismount the exam table, and I moved to allow her room to do so. She stepped right off and did not turn to back off. She walked back to her chair with a slight limp and veered to the left.

Dismount: 9.8

As she walked to her chair Carey said, "I'm less disgusted. I'll try to do as you ask, but I wish I was just myself."

"You are yourself. In fact, only the best selves can revalue themselves. This is no simple thing I ask you to do. I ask you to evolve. I ask you to adapt. It will be your hardest challenge and a testament to your truest capability," I assured her.

We hugged and I sent her out to try to live a little while she still had time to do so.

She veered to the left but still made her way down the hallway—the once gymnast with a secret past that made her able to weather the stroke that waited for her aging. The once and always Carey.

♥

Details

He would come in every four months with swelling and uncontrolled diabetes and a variable creatinine, all depending on his diet and diuretics. He kept amazing spreadsheets filled with data. Nephrologists love data, trending every little molecule in and out of channels. He would color-code the data. My heart would swell with the delicious details. He would walk me through the data. Professionally, he was an accountant and sat for hours at a desk crunching data. We got along lovingly and laughed about our addiction to data.

"1 2 2 3 2 of the 2, see," he said on this different day. He had shown up unusually late in the year, missing one follow-up surprisingly. Apparently, he had asked for the follow-up, demanded the follow-up with "the tall one." It was all he could spit out in a panic, his wife had said.

Since the last appointment, he had awoken with leg pain, growing increasingly short of breath. A long day sitting at a desk looking at numbers and suddenly blood clots and then a pulmonary embolism. In the six days he was hospitalized he developed a strange affliction. He began to say only numbers. He could not say any words. Slowly words came back but only words that he used technically at work. He was diagnosed with a stroke due to a patent foramen ovale.

In time I became "the tall one" and his wife figured out who he wanted to see. She booked the appointment, and when the day came he had so much to tell me. The faster he talked the more numbers came out. I listened, and in his numbers I understood what he was talking about, asking about. His potassium, his creatinine, his blood sugar, his blood pressure, his weight. It was incredible. He would start with a series of numbers and then I would say "your blood pressure?" Or "your weight?" Or "your blood sugar?" And he would yell, "Yes!"

Sometimes those crazy addictions create a crazy connection that can survive a bizarre twist. I wonder what would have happened if we did not look at all those spreadsheets with such zeal. What if he lost some other ability? What if he had not sat so long at the desk? What if I was not tall? What if nephrologists did not look at so many numbers with affection?

"201, 197, 215, 215, 178!"

"You were 215 pounds last I saw you and now you're 201 but you want to be 178?" I deciphered.

"Yes!" and then he sat back and sighed because someone had enthusiastically understood and embraced him. Someone was listening and speaking his language.

♥

Advance Directives

The papers had laid in a drawer beside the lingerie with a tag on still, the old pay stubs, and a half-used bottle of perfume from Duty-Free while leaving Amsterdam. As vague as time made many things, the details checked off had long been forgotten exactly. Perhaps, they were never exact to begin with.

"I appreciate that you sat down to discuss and complete the advance directives for you and your wife. I know it felt at the time a very painful discussion," I commended.

He started to tell me instead of some twenty years before. "My oldest daughter lived just down the street. We hadn't heard from her, so we walked down to check and found her murdered," he sobbed, fresh with the images. I stopped him only to let him know I did not need him to relive it all. He continued, though, trying to tell me not the scene but the aftermath. "We went with her body to the hospital to declare her dead, though she was already dead, we could see," he choked out. "While we were gone, the neighbors, who all said how sorry they were, came and robbed her and took every last thing in the house." He ground his teeth.

The weight of a twenty-year wound somehow found its way into the darkest corners of the ICU where machines pinged the lack of progress his wife was rapidly failing to make.

His wife had been admitted to the hospital with vague chest pains. She changed to vague stomach pains and had a negative cardiac workup and CT scan. Slowly her mentation deteriorated, and her abdominal pains increased diffusely. She moaned over and over, and her blood pressure dropped as she developed blood in her stool. She was transfused rapidly and the acidosis set in. As I came into her room to meet the husband and to talk about his wife needing dialysis, she arrested and I escorted him out.

As we were soon consumed by talking about his daughter's murder, a scene of surreal effort to revive his wife was playing out behind us. She was crashing swiftly, and the full authority of ten nurses and two doctors bore down on her to bring her back.

"I am sorry about how horrifying it must have been to find your daughter that way and the betrayal to feel returning to her home ransacked. I have no words for the pain in my heart after now hearing but a bit of it. I am sorry to bring you back to this moment, though, because we have to decide how we will continue, as your wife is not likely to survive this code or future ones if she can briefly return," I assessed.

His face was a mixture of foreshadowing and resolution. Somehow the decisions they made the day their daughter was murdered and her home invaded by people they called neighbors had led to an immediate decision to declare them each Do Not Resuscitate and Do Not Intubate. Somehow, they had resigned to gain back control over the uncontrollable events by declaring themselves ready to go should any events happen that invited leaving life.

The remaining daughter spoke. "They have always said to not resuscitate. Every dinner, every celebration they would announce, 'And if I die, let me go,' and we all would say we would do that."

The code carried on, and as the husband and daughter both nodded to end the affair, the wife returned and stabilized on three pressors, intubated. The window to leave closed and again we were on the brink of death.

I looked over my shoulder and saw the commotion die down, her vitals still pinging. I realized her moment to leave had left. I approached the husband again to ask if he wanted her to be dialyzed now that she was stabilized. He repeated his story about his murdered daughter, and I searched for him in the haze that had become the trauma revisited in distress.

"Sir, look at me. Are you telling me this again because you feel if I let her go it is easiest on your heart? Are you telling me this because you feel your wife is already gone? Are you telling me this because your answer about efforts to save your wife, though likely small, are like losing your daughter, only to be hurt further because it got worse after they ransacked her house?" I sought to solve the translational gap.

"My wife has already left to be with Sally," he sobbed.

To the husband, heaven's gates had been locked for twenty years, and they both had rushed to declare themselves DNR/DNI to await who would go to be with their daughter first. They arrived at conclusions so absolute that the first smell of disaster laid like a reprieve for one to leave and one to envy the release.

"Mr. Allen, I must ask you because now that we have her back as we were talking, I cannot keep her here if I don't dialyze her, but if I don't try after she has come back, I fear in a short time you will be left with guilt that you gave up. I do not know that if I try, she will even tolerate it, but I need to painfully ask you how you want this narrative to retell. To strangers, months from now or to yourself alone without her in the dark at 2 a.m., do you want to say you did all you could and even then it was not working?" I asked the drawn-out version that the Advance Directives could never delineate in a time that can never be fully experienced to check a box and declare it decided in advance.

"The papers said to do everything unless she is terminal," he reviewed as if every night before bed they had said it together out loud as a promise.

"Mr. Allen, she is likely terminal, but she is also young, still here, and needing more support if you can permit the placement of the dialysis catheter and to start dialysis. I am sorry to continue to discuss this as if I am daft. I need to know because she can code again while we discuss or soon after while I make arrangements. I do not have much time, so I just need you to tell me things that tell me if you will be okay to proceed or not to proceed." I struggled to pressure him and to get from him clear direction that honored their intentions.

"Do it. But my wife has already gone to Sally," he said, firm and sorrowful.

I took what truth I could use out of his statement with witnesses around and began to order the needed interventions. He hovered around the nurses' station, not sure where to stand or sit. I hugged him but he did not hug back, and I left to discuss the case with others.

In a few hours of starting dialysis gently, she coded again, and he let them work on her for ten minutes before he commanded them to stop. The team seemed baffled by the early cease, but so many attempts at embolizing intestinal bleeding unsuccessfully stayed as evidence of futility.

The dialysis stopped and blood was returned, and her vitals pinged a few last beats, then had to be silenced for all the alarms went off with hostility and vengeance like a horn blowing the gates of Heaven open for her.

"My wife has gone to be with my daughter," the husband reassured himself and us. Those who knew the sorrowful details of a murdered daughter knew the painful closure, and those who did not know merely saw the vagueness of the statement.

♥

The Sun We Rise

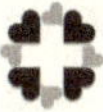

"I thought," she panted, "I would live to ninety-five like my mom, but—" She pushed on with the oxygen hissing. "—here I am at eighty-three, dying."

I watched her chest ebb up and down declaring a respiratory rate of thirty-six breaths per minute. I realized my mother was a real and fallible person when she was thirty-six years old. My thoughts spun around dividing 36 by 6 and adding 10 randomly and then I glanced to see her on six liters of oxygen with three tubes coming out of her body. Time then was an entity in the room I had to address.

"I had a mortal moment once when I was thirty-six," I told her. "I always thought I would live to eighty-nine, but my arthritis made me consider the reality I wasn't going to live to eighty-nine or at best I might but I would cross the finish line maybe in a wheelchair, a burden on someone behind me pushing. My point," I begged her for consideration, "is though these thoughts are natural and important, let them go. You are so very short on time."

She released her hold on vanity.

"I lived such a great—" She pursed her lips. "—life. I had a husband who respected me and stood by my side. I had great children and a purpose. I just want to lie by my Sam in bed."

The room filled with her new, meatier thoughts. "See," I announced, "those thoughts are full and beefy with life. Focus on those. Share those. Those are the words your sacred breaths should be used on now. Your family should hear these thoughts." I urged her to gift them to the family on their way in. These thoughts would feed her loved ones after she had passed for a lifetime.

She nodded with unusual effort so short of breath and we said goodbyes. I hated to leave her but her breaths were too precious a commodity in a room full of things to waste on me chatting, and though she was dying, a death watch would scare her, so I left, head bowed, crying and not so softly. I had met her only two days earlier, and at first glance of her pale skin and lip quiver, I could tell she already was extinguishing too fast. I fell in love with her composure; I faced the dilemma of making a friend who was leaving soon.

Worried over her transition, I came back. The two youngest children were there, and I introduced myself. She was unconscious. "Did you just get in?" I wondered, anxious to know.

"Yeah, just an hour ago," the daughter replied without excruciating heartache but instead with enough salve applied. I hoped they had arrived with her still talking.

"Was she awake when you came?" I inched into a cold pool of sorrow.

"No."

The room shrank, and all the meaty things oozed out of the pie and onto the counter. I panicked and pleaded in my breaths, now matching hers at forty a minute. I even closed my eyes to find her better.

"Ugh," I groaned and sighed, "she had told me some things I had told her to tell you all and her husband Sam. I, uh, I need to tell them to you because I cannot be the one to have heard it last."

They eagerly accepted my invitation, and as their visit closed, they took me to find their father and eldest brother.

We gathered in front of the hospital in the parking lot.

"It was the way she came about these words. It was how she is leaving all this. She was at first thinking of disappointing realities. I told her that time was too short to ponder meaningless things. She immediately listened and turned to be grateful." I shared her last words to me and the emotion of being self-pleased with respect from a husband and with pride in watching children bloom. "And she just wanted to lie in bed with you, sir. She called you Sam so sweetly it made me feel her falling in love," I told her husband of sixty-three years.

Then the gentle wind came, a contrast to her halted and shallow breaths. "Thank you for telling us this." They kept composure. "She told us this so often and so clearly," they assured me so I had been certainly accurate.

"That," I prickled, "is the best realization of a well-lived and loved life. I thought I would give back to you her last thoughts and assure you her peace in transition, but *you* give me insight that her last words were hers, *always* in her heart and on her lips. What a person she was to teach how to pass without the climax of unspoken and unknown things. May she live forever in your already full and constant awareness of her and her intentions of you four. Remarkable. I wish I had longer around someone like her."

I parted, returning back to the hospital, wondering if I could leave life today uttering no other words left unsaid in a thick trust that my loved ones already knew my last thoughts, wants, and thanks. Vain only as a trademark of being human, I hoped to die one day silent because I had said it all while living.

♥

Passive Torture

He had extreme motion sickness and chose to ride only with his wife, who worked the days she could in between his appointments. During the time I cared for him, when he switched doctors so as to "not be yelled at," he had only several great weeks of compliance, attending each dialysis session fully.

"Wow! What a great two weeks! Do you feel better?" I hoped.

"Yeah . . . I do," he hesitated. Though he remained openly unable to promise me "a change of character," we delighted to give him an "Honor Roll" certificate anyway for his efforts. Immediately after the award was given, he started missing treatments again. The dietitian missed him several times to explain our selection and eventually was left feeling a bit silly to have awarded a fleeting moment.

"I almost gave up trying to see him to explain the whole 'Honor roll' certificate," she confessed. She finally caught up with him one day and boosted his prior success, hoping to reignite his efforts.

I gathered he avoided me, sometimes not coming to dialysis when he knew I would be there. When we would chance meet, he negotiated every term, and the tone of his voice when involved plans were discussed said to me he was not long for this world of effort. There were many goals he could not achieve without more than two steps back, and he seemed to draw lines in the sand to say if it came to such realities of long-involved dominoes he would forfeit. Once, he and his wife came to my office for privacy and a "powwow." He struggled to commit then to any plans. I merely offered the plans to choose from with descriptions of the consequential fates for each. I was never frustrated or judgmental. I gave him the reins of accountability but gauged that he was gruff because he saw fear.

"I just want," his wife added, "more anniversaries with you."

This declaration was the highlight of that meeting, and we rode the ramifications of such a plea like a wave promising inspirational change. He picked the moderate plan and aimed to achieve it. The wave crashed onto the beach, and the tide fell back into the motion sickness of living on dialysis with barely the will to commit to the rigors of boating in the ocean.

He flirted with death constantly for the year we engaged, and he changed just so slightly. His whole family and I saw that slight change as his rebirth.

Finally, the potassium was reportedly lethal, for which he refused hospitalization. I panicked to get him to understand and pleaded with him to "please go to the hospital." He did not go, and two days later he arrived instead to the unit and did not stay but twenty minutes into a 3.5-hour treatment, and so I knew he was passively exiting.

I called his wife, who was now fully in charge because he was beginning to be uremic and confused. Wasted and fragile, he lay in bed while she and I decided.

"It is time," I permitted.

She agreed, though she wanted badly for him to declare it.

"He is declaring it passively," I reassured. "Not all can say they are ready, but therein lies the responsibility you have. I will own too in hearing what he is truly saying."

I had my staff make arrangements for hospice. Twenty-four hours after he enrolled, I got the call that he had passed.

I called his wife soon after. "I'm sorry he was tortured," I said.

"He was tortured, but in the end he was freed. He did tell me he was ready at the end," his wife said, relieved. I was glad for her release. It is hard to be the one left and the one eternally responsible. There is no peace inside for the living who doubt every last decision and lack of persuasion even if that was never the narrative. The mind seems to twist the past to torture the living in lies.

"I'm grateful for that closure," I sighed, heavy with relief.

"You know, he came home one day telling me he had made Honor Roll," she laughed.

My heart lit up like a Fourth of July firecracker, and I raced to tell her our secret joy.

"You know," I shared, "we sit around each month and do a lot of logistical analysis to make sure our quality of care is on task. It rededicates us to the novelty of encouraging people. Then at the end, we take great pleasure in awarding our patients' efforts and individual success. We literally discuss the unique accomplishment and reasons for celebrations for their personal achievements. Seeing your husband try even parts of what I asked made me so proud," I beamed.

"Thank you for giving him some dignity in the last year of his life," she expressed.

"It was my pleasure," I returned.

Upon hanging up with her, I called the dietitian, who was in cahoots with me to champion patients.

"I wanted you to know it mattered, and I appreciate your efforts and enthusiasm. Thank you for handing out the certificates," I shared.

Let us lead this fight with dignity and wisdom, finding dignity and wisdom for all. Let us find the peace that stays and invite life to feed forward despite the seeming torture living can become.

♥

Sunset Skin

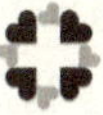

It was an election year. Everything sounded like propaganda. I worried that my passion for narratology would be laughed out and betray me when others claimed it was nothing but parlor tricks and overthinking a simple design.

"Well, that's just good medicine," the bioethicist seemed to maintain about the impact of Narrative Medicine as a unique discipline, and the words would crush a little fledgling idea that had seemed to shine a little light in a darkening and musty space.

But stories kept unfolding.

He was lying in an ICU bed like a zigzag. His puffy mittens and thin sheet thrown over his body seemed like a disheveled-looking afterthought by his writhing. I felt dismayed, like I had opened a present to find a broken vase. I pulled back part of the sheet to examine his yellow skin and saw large purple bruises in saucer-sized patches all over his legs and abdomen. He moaned a bit as I pressed my stethoscope on his chest. His lips were dry, and I felt the pain of the cracked skin.

The nurse entered the room. She knew me well. She started by looking where my gaze was, and we met, looking up from the same person plopped down on the bed as if to leave him on some sidewalk.

She started because she knew me to need the narrative.

"His mother, poor thing, told us she found him on the floor. He is a Veteran and he just lost his dog, who was everything to him. He has no wife or kids, just the dog. He had a lot of PTSD, but the medications they gave him made him so sleepy he just stopped taking them. He started drinking more and using some drugs and, well, he would be at his house doing yardwork and drinking outside. His mother said she couldn't seem to help him and would go by to check on him, always worried what she would find," she laid out.

"Hmmm," I nodded, taking in the person and the journey that led to a lost dog spiraling a lonely young man into a bruised abyss. His liver agonized along with him, and the mortality score cast a grim sentence of three months.

"He just lost the dog and well gave up." The nurse busied herself telling the man it was okay when he groaned and straightened his wrangled sheet.

"I hope he wakes up calm but I fear he will wake up in a frantic whirlpool of emotions, not knowing why he is here and what is going on. I hope he wakes and gets to choose what he wants from these near misses that aren't actually near misses. He can't wake up from a more important nightmare," I contemplated.

The nurse knew I was interested in his narrative. I could not find a peaceful exit, and she understood the conflict. "The system fails these Veterans," she reflected. "You should see the mother and sister. They are so relieved he is here."

"The hospital is a safe haven for a short time, but then what?" I worried. I left the room waiting to see if he would wake in the next days and what way his needs would lean toward. How much could we really do as we set him back to spinning when he was well enough to leave the hospital? It was the yellowed sky once hopeful now blemished with purple clouds that seemed agitated and bruting, worn as his skin, that I could not stop feeling ashamed about. I was not brave enough or physical enough to join the military. Yet here was our war and war story, come to take safe haven for a spell.

"Thank you for telling me things that matter about him. I really appreciate that insight and you for finding it out," I thanked the nurse.

It was an election year and many opinions are floated about what is worth the time, money, and effort. Regardless, medicine remained the same: people caring for people every day with stories to be shared.

♥

Taking the Other Road

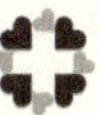

"You know what? I got my year-end evaluation and a parent wrote 'mediocre teacher, just in it for the money,'" she suddenly shared.

"What the . . . What does that even mean?!" I replied, half burning with offense and half dumbfounded with confusion because teachers make scraps and she volunteered so much of her own time. "What money are you 'in it for'?" I asked, seething with swear words in my head. She was a very intelligent and methodical teacher who grew her students fundamentally over a year's time. She matured them in all ways and never spared the rod or a hug. It was easy for me to see her love for the children and her philosophy. It was heartwarming to feel her thoughtfulness, and I found her incredible. I trusted her with my own child, and my child bloomed. We became friends over time, and I respected her as a colleague against ignorance, a maker of betterment, a fellow farmer of citizens.

"I know! I don't even swear, and I just read that and out came, 'What the fuck?!' It makes me cry. I feel so defeated," she admitted. Her shoulders slumped and her voice lowered. "Not too long ago I was pre-med." She fought back tears.

I usually encounter a lot of people saying they "were pre-med" like it is a badge of some half-baked achievement with a weight of practically achieved. Frustrated and low on self-esteem, people try to defend themselves contesting the possibility of a path almost traveled. Yet, she wasn't defending herself quite the same. She wasn't trying to inflate herself. I didn't feel like I had to humor her.

"I was everything. Dozens of advance placement credits, all my prerequisites. I took the MCAT and did great. Then . . ." She stopped to cry and began to hiccup.

I saw her at a fork in the road. I saw myself go one way and her go the other road. I saw her sad to choose.

"People don't know. They don't know that Bill then got Stage 4 lymphoma and we just had to adjust everything. Deeds was a baby, and I needed a job and to be home. I needed to still love what I did but I just needed to stop climbing my own ambition or I would lose Bill and Deeds wouldn't have a daddy." She had gutted her own ego.

I stood corrected universally. She opened my eyes to the many untold stories. I began to realize some of the most qualified applicants looking to join medicine must take the other road. Some of our sisters and brothers must go on a different path, and they should go with our support to other destinations. But they say the gifted can see each other well and identify the fire that burns within. They say the gifted merely circle around to each other and share the larger journey afoot. Divide and conquer. Even within medicine we must often take what we think are lesser roads. We move forward down roads we did not plan for with shame and sadness. Why? We are no less the warrior.

Being a doctor is not for all. For some very driven, very capable, it cannot be. For some it asks too much.

"You are not mediocre," I declared.

She dried her tears. "It just hurts that someone would say this, and I wonder which child I failed, which parent I failed." She painfully bore raw on her chest these self-doubts.

"You didn't fail anyone," I maintained. "You are as capable and as effective as you would've been in another role, and even more sacredly you are 'doctoring' children toward healthy adult lives. Never doubt yourself. You have great gifts to give. There will always be others who will try to rob dedication and ability with meaningless and 'mediocre' words," I winked. "What does that statement even mean except that an idiot spoke it, confusing terms and truths and ideas?"

She nodded. "You're so kind," she thanked.

"Actually, I'm ruthlessly critical. I'm not patronizing you. You are a very respectable teacher. I would never discount you for not being a doctor. That is not our sisterhood. Ours is above description and title. I just see you as a passionate person excelling. Mediocre people don't cry at being called mediocre," I justified.

She wiped her tears and stood a little taller. The insult faded a bit against the recalling of terms that made her take the other road. She would spend her life teaching critical things at critical moments in a child's life. Life imitates medicine, and living is medicinal.

♥

Left to Do

Months ago, she brought her husband into my office. She wanted me to "tell him," so I "told him" everything.

"I don't understand," he quivered. "I don't understand," he repeated. "There isn't anything you can do?"

"No," I exhaled.

It had been an arduous and torturous delineation of the end game for pulmonary hypertension. Her concentrator sucked and hummed its six liters in the background of heavy footfalling sentences.

She knew the heavier words between the lines and yet he repeated, "I don't understand. There's nothing?"

"No." I drew a flat blanket over a beaten notion's face and proclaimed it a dead matter.

They left that day with him shaking his head without understanding. He might have hated me a bit except it was hard to hate someone who hugged him.

Today the patient fridge was fresh out of Jell-O. I fancied a Jell-O, but there was only vanilla pudding. I grabbed two containers. They were icebox cold in my hand. I grabbed two spoons sleeved in protective plastic and headed to a room that mirrored the other twenty on the pod. I entered her room and looked upon a man's long face. My eyes dropped down in the deepest of sympathy, and I reached out my free hand to firmly shake his. He knew me right away.

I came around to his bride of fifty-two years lying in bed at ninety degrees, eyes closed and breathing heavily. "Mrs. Houston. Mrs. Houston," I stirred. Perhaps I was too late. Her eyes blinked open and she focused after a few seconds on my face. "Dr. Robey?" she chanced in disbelief. "You're here?" she smiled weakly.

"I thought we could have some pudding together. Sometimes we break bread and sometimes we break pudding," I joked and peeled back a pudding flap. She smacked her dry lips a bit, appearing interested or at least socially graceful at my hosting.

"If she can eat some I would be so happy," her loving husband shifted.

I spooned a bit up into a spoon and she opened her mouth gently. She took the very cold and very creamy dollop into her mouth and let its coolness slide down her dried throat. "Mmmm," she thanked.

"Would you like one, sir?" I offered her husband.

"Well, if you have two there that sounds just right." He reached. I handed him the pudding twin and a personally packaged spoon. It was like snack time for youth again. I continued to feed her slowly, just two more bites, as her husband ate all of his.

"Look at you two eating like love birds together. So romantic," I teased as she smacked the third bite of cold, refreshing thoughts and laughed.

"You are the nicest person," she said. "Thank you. Just . . ." She gasped a little. "Thank you."

Her husband put the empty container down, wiped respectfully clean like a gourmet brûlée.

"I keep the best company by being nice." I winked at her. "Please let us know if you need anything. God is with you. He has given you good company," and I kissed her cheek softly goodbye.

"Thank you for coming." He nodded from the porch of our ice tea time together.

"Yes, sir. There was, after all, this one more thing I found I could do," I realized.

♥

Thank You for Your Referral

He arrived a very shy, polite man. One eye laid lazily shut. He answered all questions agreeably as I typed.

"Who sent you to me?" I inquired, hoping to gleam a piece of matter that would create the universal quilt.

"Dr. Johnson," he replied. "I'm not," he confessed, "sure why?"

My inner eye winked across the city to my friend whom I knew weighed a person for all their needs, and there I began the puzzle with this cornerstone detail.

He got up on the table and I examined him. In between my hands moving from organ systems, I asked questions. "Do you have children?"

"A stepson," he answered, "in California."

I regarded the mention of a stepson as meaning no children of his own. I regarded the state away that kept them apart too.

"No children of your own," I clarified, standing at his profile.

His lazy eye opened a bit wider, and he inhaled to explain. "A year before I met my wife she had a hysterectomy. She gave me a choice . . . and I chose her."

How he answered my point of clarity made my heart swell. Here was a man in love.

"Do you get out much? Have friends?" I asked, running my hands into his armpits and neckline.

"Acquaintances," he chagrined. "Well," he continued, "when Nancy was sick, they came by but then . . . stopped. I know it's hard to be around people who are sick . . . people get sick! Anyway, they are just acquaintances."

It broke my swollen heart to hear the pain of abandonment in his voice.

I helped him off the table and brushed my hand on his wedding band.

His wife had died nineteen months ago. So, here we were.

"Okay. Let me offer you three things," I said. "First, your kidneys are filters and they are not normal but are not bad. You have Stage 3 disease, and in this stage we focus on managing all your medical contributors. These are all perfectly managed." I filled the cold cup with facts and details as advertised upon referral. It was quickly done. He was satisfied. We could have ended it there.

"Secondly, you are here for something much more, if you allow me," I asked. He permitted me some latitude. "You have said exquisite things. I know Dr. Johnson cares for you and that you must be one of her favorites to have sent you here. This is not a pat on my back. It is an admission of my little value toward your kidney health. It is more a reflection that you are in need of TLC. Dr. Johnson knows I do TLC."

He laughed and it encouraged me to continue. "You are stuck somewhere, and I am to help you get unstuck. Thus, thirdly, you need help to find this detail. I will need your help to do so. I believe you are still very sad, very in love, very lonely. I think . . . I think you need to find friends, and forgive these other friends who seemed to have failed you, to begin to live again."

The man sat shocked and raised his left hand to show me his wedding band. "I cannot bear to take it off," he wept.

"Sir—" I wiped my eyes under my glasses for the glare of beauty was so intense. "—let me tell you what you said to me just now. You said, 'A year before we met she had a hysterectomy and gave me a choice and

I chose her.' You said 'acquaintances' like a bitter taste in your throat, choking back a lump covered by a salty tear. Sir, you have sorrow and these friends you hoped would have your back let you down while you and your wife suffered. I know you love your wife. I know. Can I give you a gift?"

He nodded.

"My friend and I have been speaking of friends, friends who disappoint. Then we realized there may be many other ways to define friends. Maybe there's a definition of a friend who is still a friend to bring joy or levity. Could you find these types of friends, or renew relationships on new terms? Could these friends and friendships make some new life for you? Isn't it time?"

He mused at these thoughts and accepted the gift of daring perspective.

"We used to play bocci ball," he replied.

"Yes, yes . . ." I lured him out to fill the blanks in my general surmises.

"They were good friends," he smiled.

"Yes, keep talking," I coaxed.

"Fun," he added.

I leaned in eagerly. "Well, they invited me after Nancy died but I . . . I don't know," he hesitated.

"Let's do this!" I gambled. "Let's say the last group was a couples thing, but now that we have been gone let's go back as a singlet and remake ourselves!"

He smiled and nodded and the lazy lid lit up.

"There's a couple that did stand by us. They come in October from Washington . . . the husband and I get a burger sometimes," he shared.

"Awesome! Let's call him for sure!" I riveted.

He sat up and forward, and his aura glimmered into clarity. "Well," I reflected, looking him over as if his face had peered up from a muddy pond, "there you are."

The man awoke out of a nineteen-month slumber and was now sparkling. "You're such a pleasure to meet. Did you forget that?" I teased.

He smiled, and we both rose as he readied to leave. "Thank you for coming. It has been a wonderful visit, sir."

"I think you're right. I think Dr. Johnson was right. I think I understand why Dr. Johnson sent me here," he assessed. "She was so good to Nancy and now me."

"She sent you because she loves you," I agreed. "She likely loved you both."

Dear Dr. Johnson,

I met a patient of yours today. He was an amazing treat. Thank you for sending him.

Sincerely,
Jean

♥

Bearer of Bad News

Nowadays I am asked to interview applicants for medical school and residency programs. It is an honor to engage and evaluate these potential candidates. It means being entrusted with a kind of vision for the profession's future, but more tangibly it means a perspective that is looking essentially for the candidates that will be basically *my* own physician one day. Who will doctor me, literally, as I age, and how will they deliver news good and bad at the bedside?

He was awake complaining about pain but calm and conversant. His elective surgery had very unexpected complications. A planned aortic graft became a rapid dissection and then an ischemic right leg. He was able to be extubated after the procedure, seemingly stabilized, but the tissues in the leg were dying and the pain was rising up his leg, knee, thigh, and groin and into his whole soul and throat. The release of toxic elements and electrolytes rapidly shut down his kidneys and short-circuited the neurohormonal feedbacks that helped to maintain blood pressure. His last clear thoughts were focused on me telling him what was happening and the multitude of things to expect including intubation and kidney failure. I left off the need for a heroic effort of cutting off his leg, and he drifted into unconsciousness as we stabilized him by reintubating him.

"Hello, is this Mrs. Jones?" I rang after I was able to pull away.

"Yes," her voice trembled. "It is."

She was in the waiting room and met me in the hallway to discuss the events and the current state of affairs. She looked weakened with each slay of details, and the summary nailed a blow to her chest that made her reach up and place her hand on her bosom. I motioned her to a chair, and she sat with her face falling into her hands as she wept.

"He is getting stabilized now, but I have to ask you about whether he would agree to dialysis to help stabilize him and explain the risks and benefits. I will tell you that cases like this need to have very radical efforts that include amputation of the leg," I pushed.

She wept and I let her. The air around her crowded in and hugged her, then with each sob the air expanded outward to make space. After a minute I apologized. "I am sorry to keep going. I wish I could stop." Her emotional exhaustion weighed down the dust around us, and all that walked passed entered the haboob. She pulled her hands away from her sobbing face and tried to focus.

"I can't imagine him waking with no leg," she concluded.

I sat down at that comment and held her hands and tried to be her then, be him, and then tried to be him waking with no leg. She had a specific reason to say what she said, and I held my breath against the acidity of time to hear it.

"He is a hunter. He loves to go hunting. That is why we did this surgery, to help him be active and go hunting safely. He cannot go hunting if he has no leg," she explained.

I pressed, "Do you think he would overcome such an outcome and get a prosthesis?"

"No. He never wanted to be like that. He had friends in the Vietnam War and they had these prosthetics and he just felt their life was so compromised. He has told me so many times till I yelled confused, 'Why do you talk about having no leg or arm?' He told me so clearly he would never choose to go on like that."

The oddness of the prophecy hung in the air. At sixty-nine years old, Mr. Jones lay in the wasteland of medicine, trying and not trying. The hardship we would impose amputating his leg would subject him to the potential of inevitable failure as he might lose the will to compromise a much held decree.

"Is there any chance you would regret not trying?" I pushed.

"He just . . . so clearly told me till I was just so angry, he was like obsessed with making sure I knew how he felt," she contemplated.

I left the grieving wife. She had sat in the waiting room waiting for news that she could take her husband home to recuperate in a few days, and now in hours she was facing a reality that rapidly meant absolute decisions to do absolute things that would be life, death, or a hell on Earth her husband had avoided in war but predicted and overemphasized in peacetime. There would be no negotiations as he was unconscious, but ironically they had already been denied so many times before when a hypothetical. I informed the team and left the last line of my note: "Please call with any change in status."

The next morning very early, I checked to see how the conversations had evolved and found that Mr. Jones had passed. The care had escalated over an hour, and he was very tenuous, but the wife with her son by her side decided to let go and withdraw. The wife fulfilled her obligation to execute her husband's wishes to not leave him legless and let go.

"So," I ask the applicant these days, "how do you feel about giving bad news and feeling conflict and going home with feelings of conflict?"

The air becomes unsure as to the real nature of the question or the real value of the self-exploration. The man with two legs, the man with one leg, the wife alone, the wife with the son by the side, the hunter, the intubated to never wake again, the man who came for elective surgery but left the world as we know it for endless skies, the doctor huddled in a hallway speechless and later checking the chart for the way a story ends, all coexist in the air as the question tries to find the future bearer of the torch to guide.

♥

Appointment Cancellation

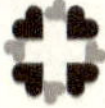

Dear Dr. Robey.

I had to cancel my last appointment since I had a slight fever & now I have to cancel this one on the 9th.

I'm going through a tough time. My husband passed away recently & I'm in a difficult situation.

My feet have been swollen for weeks and I can't wear shoes. I no longer have family here and I know my kidney's are the problem, but I refuse to go on dialysis. I'm on 8 meds, I'm diabetic, have osteoporosis, severe neuropathy & can't sit too long because of the pain

I have to get up & walk for a minute which I could not do in the hospital. I spend most of the day with my feet elevated and do what I can but having 3 cousins on dialysis convinced me not to spend my last days like that.

I have good neighbors that help but some are snowbirds.

I know since you're a doctor you may feel obligated to try to help & it's not your fault I refuse. I'll be 88 soon so I'll live with my choice.

Appointment Cancellation:

Student Reflection by Jade Robey, University of Arizona College of Medicine—Tucson, Class 2029

Patients can feel stripped of their choices when they find themselves conflicted and alone in unnavigable territory. In spaces meant for healing, autonomy can feel like the first casualty. Doctors, armed with knowledge and clinical solutions, can feel all-knowing when presented with a patient. There is truth in knowing what the next best medical steps are, and there is truth in the art of medicine, in understanding what cannot be found on a chart or in laboratory results but in the quiet confessions of a patient who has weighed suffering against dignity and has told the physician their story.

After reading this letter, I did not feel confused or conflicted or even sad. I felt clarity. All I could feel was a clear understanding of the life of this patient and their decision, and a certain happiness that they had the courage to decide what meant more to them than suffering and fighting for the last of their physical health. I understood the loss of a husband and the restraint of a hospital room. I felt the shackles of swollen ankles unfit for shoes or much walking and the contradictory pain from sitting too long. I felt guilty that there was anticipation of conflict from my mother, this patient's doctor and ally, that she might push them to do something that did not align with their reality.

Seated in an uncomfortable chair because nothing is truly comfortable anymore, I saw the patient writing in the most beautiful cursive a letter part confession, part declaration, part apology. I pictured my mother's patient wanting to let their doctor know that they did not fail their duties, but in truth, it was the complexity of their reality that dared to dismantle the system built upon simplified, idealized patient goals. The real patient had lived a life shaped by loss, immobility, and exhaustion and could not be reduced to theory and warrant a visit to a meager illusion of a buffet of betterment. The true measure of care instantly became not just in offering solutions but in honoring the deeply human narratives that make each patient's experience uniquely their own. The value of reading her story strung out in elegant flowing cursive rather than reading a chart became part testament to honoring narratives while doctoring most effectively.

♥

Afterword
Why Using a Coaching Approach Is Important

By Marcia Reynolds, PsyD, MCC

My first master's degree was in Broadcast Communication, which earned me the important job of pushing television sets and film projectors around three hospitals. I reported to the training department. Eventually, I was included in creating and delivering training programs. My focus shifted to learning about what inspires sustainable change. I remember two significant facts.

1) You can tell people they will die if they don't follow a specific protocol. They will comply, for a short period of time, until they rationalize they don't need to completely comply or not at all. Some die. And the smarter a person is, the better they are at rationalizing behavior.

2) The relationship with the health professional—if they felt seen, heard, and a full human—had a lot to do with their trust that what was prescribed should be followed. Fear was not the major motivator. They needed to feel the physician, assistant, or nurse practitioner sincerely

cared about them, with sincerity being an energetic exchange beyond the spoken word.

After years of studying adult learning, I found the best way to address both of these facts was with coaching. Telling people what to do may elicit short-term change, but sustainable change requires a shift in perspective that can be achieved through coaching with reflective inquiry, sharing stories as metaphors, and poetry reading and writing where strong emotions spark creative insights. After meeting Dr. Jean Robey, I discovered this type of doctoring aligns with Narrative Medicine.

My expertise and passion is in coaching where we act as the person's thinking partner instead of the expert with power over them. When we act as thinking partners, we can break through old thinking patterns to create new ideas, foster emotional commitment, and ensure mental development.

Professor Carin Eriksson Lindvall at Uppsala University said humans don't change habits and behaviors even when they have experienced undesirable results; most routines are disturbed for only a short time or not changed at all. Between letting go and trying to behave a new way is a foggy, unmarked path. Our brains don't like and then resist the state of "not knowing." The brain then prefers to stay home.

People usually don't change even when they know they should. Their brains choose self-preservation over self-care.

Psychologist Dan McAdams of Northwestern University says old goals, obsolete values, and outdated beliefs about what is right and wrong provide a sense of consistency. We all become master rationalizers to avoid the discomfort of change.

This is why giving advice is the least effective way to change someone's mind. They may hear you and agree to try something new, but as soon as an attempt to change feels awkward, they will rationalize going back to old beliefs and behaviors.

We need "external thought disruptors" when the desired outcome is for people to act differently than they do today. To see differently, your patients need someone else to compassionately reflect their words and expressions and ask questions that stop the automatic processing. Neuroscientist Michael Gazzangia maintained that if a person has an external though disruptor—someone to summarize key words spoken and express emotions, asking about meaning and importance in the moment, then they can expand their comfort zone. Disruptors also patiently and lovingly share spoken contradictions and call out what beliefs seem to be the source of hesitations so these thoughts can be objectively observed and analyzed.

An external thought disrupter overrides the protective brain with these concise reflective statements—summaries of words shared and emotions expressed—followed by gentle, curious questions. The insights disrupt their brain's operating system. They can then "see" their thoughts and beliefs outside of the brain and more objectively consider what thoughts, beliefs, and fears are directing decisions and actions today, and what they might now believe is the best course of action for them. They might also develop more confidence in procedures and the strength to endure complications.

Once patients see their narratives on display, they can recognize and accept the gaps in logic, the outdated beliefs, the unsupported assumptions, and the "shoulds" keeping them from moving toward their more desired outcome. Using a respectful coaching approach breaks through the frames holding their old stories together. Only then can perceptions of the situation and oneself begin to shift.

Educational reformer John Dewey said, "Provoking people to think about their thinking is the single most powerful antidote to erroneous beliefs and autopilot." Reality is persistent, but coaching can create the breakthroughs where the emerging insights expand what is possible for all humans we encounter.

I am so passionate about the impact coaching can have to expand consciousness, strengthen professional and personal relationships, and uplift spirits in our chaotic world that I have written a number of books on the transformative experience of coaching. I teach and adhere to the skills defined as active coaching competencies, but I believe the effectiveness of coaching skills depends on the depth and richness of coaching mindset and presence.

When working to develop presence with caring patience and compassionate curiosity, you don't have to be a trained coach to use a coaching approach that breaks through someone's automatic rationalizing and imaginary outcomes. If you feel curious based on a sincere desire to understand how a person thinks, your presence soothes their fear of judgment. They sense you are there for their higher good and may feel safe enough to respond to the reflections you share and the questions you ask. You trigger oxytocin so they bond with you and serotonin, which deepens their trust. Even if there are moments of hesitation or resistance, if you don't negatively react to their emotions, their mental fog will clear enough to see a step they can take toward achieving their desired outcomes and goals.

Even if you simply summarize their spoken thoughts and then ask questions about what their words mean, they will respond more positively than if you just tell them what you have found and what they should then do. Maintaining your presence and curiosity is more important than being smart and profound. Your caring curiosity provides the safety they need to accept a new reality and commit to their best care.

Developing emotional intelligence is also key to maintaining a safe and trusting conversation. The first time a person sees with unfiltered clarity how their behavior and decisions have impacted their past experiences can be upsetting. A painful realization is a healthy part of the process. Discomfort is evidence that a new awareness is forming. Allowing their reactions to exist and then subside without jumping in to fix them or ease their pain will sustain the partnership needed for the transformation to unfold.

When you give people a moment to process what they now see with kindhearted silence, their emotional reaction will subside. When you sense they are settling down, you can ask them if they would share what they now see. Painful, embarrassing, and heart-wrenching realizations may be inevitable, but with coaching, most people feel lighter and optimistic after experiencing a new awareness and talking through what the new awareness means to them.

Presence is not an action. Coaching presence is a positive dynamic state of energy that forms and maintains the connection between two people throughout their conversations. The person being coached feels respected and cared about, and that the focus of the conversation is for their benefit and not someone else's agenda. Coaching mindset and presence will increase or decrease the acceptance of the coaching skills used.

Once the energetic bond is established, the critical coaching skills for leaders to learn include

- Using compassionate curiosity
- Responding with empathy
- Exploring meaning and desired outcomes with reflective inquiry
- Identifying limiting beliefs, assumptions, and conflicts of values
- Evoking awareness with stories and metaphors
- Ensuring a commitment to act

I believe all conversations would benefit from using a coaching approach. Even in conflict situations, we can come together to find a suitable way forward. Using a coach approach in our conversations can help us rise above the chaos in the world. And with how medicine is changing, Narrative Medicine using coach-like skills facilitates the unique and important relationships in medicine that shape true wellness.

Marcia Reynolds, PsyD, MCC
May 2025

♥

About the Author

Jean Robey has been a practicing nephrologist in Arizona since 2006. She is an Arizona Flinn Scholar Class of 1992 and a graduate of the University of Arizona College Medicine in Tucson as a Dean Scholar. She attended the Medical University of South Carolina for Surgical Internship, Internal Medicine Residency, and Nephrology Fellowship. She is a professor of Narrative Medicine, Internal Medicine, and Nephrology. She mentors prospects to medicine and medical students seeking residency training. She is now section leader for the Department of Nephrology at an Internal Medicine residency program in Surprise, Arizona. She writes prose and poetry and her work has led to collaborations with multiple artist. In November 2025, her collaboration with local artist Marshall Shore @hiphistorian through an opportunity with Artist + Researcher Phoenix (ARx) will be on exhibit at the Arizona Science Center. This exhibit will be a artistic rendition of Narrative Medicine. Her hope is to bring Narrative Medicine through her stories into broader light as a coachable practice for physicians in training and to address burnout for established physicians given the inevitable burnout that comes with decades of practicing medicine with deep commitment. To the greater audience, she hopes the stories will provide insight, validation, and a kind of goalpost for intimate physician-patient encounters.

"She looked at me like no one had ever listened or loved her before," wrote Dr. Robey.

When not running around busy addressing medically complex problems, Dr. Robey enjoys traveling, cruising, cooking, reading, playing with her pets, and getting together with family. She and her husband Kirk have called Arizona their forever home. She is extremely proud of her family's evolution after arriving in America and of her children's future born of that opportunity.

Request for Reviews

Thank you for joining me in the exam rooms and lives of people like yourself. Would you do me a favor?

I rely on online reviews to encourage others to read and practice to preserve the best parts of doctoring and patient engagements. Your opinion is invaluable to inspire future leaders in medicine to join the narrative and to train them in the art of narrative doctoring. Would you take a few moments now to share your assessment of my book at the review site of your choice? Your opinion will resist the growing singularity of medicine and help connect all who are unseen, unheard, and unknown.

Thank you very much!

May you find a caring physician enthralled in you story who adds accurate and meaningful discernment.

Be well,
Dr. Jean Robey

www.ingramcontent.com/pod-product-compliance
Lightning Source LLC
Chambersburg PA
CBHW030514130726
47901CB00013B/529

9798999956804